An Analytical Approach To Women's Health In Fertility Of Reproductive Communicable Diseases

Patrick

a) Ultrasound (US):

One of the key techniques for early PCOS prediction is ultrasound imaging of the ovary. Around the time of the first menstrual cycle of puberty, PCOS signs and symptoms often start to manifest. PCOS, for instance, might appear later in life as a consequence of severe weight gain (Di Michele et al., 2025).**Transvaginal Ultrasound (TV-US)** is considered to be the gold standard for adults. TV-US provides superior resolution, allowing detailed visualization of ovarian follicles and volume (van der Ham et al., 2025). **Transabdominal ultrasound is** utilized when TV-US is not feasible, such as in adolescents or women with limited pelvic access. **Imaging is ideally performed during the early follicular phase (days 3-5) of the menstrual cycle to avoid confusion with a dominant follicle** or the corpus luteum. There are some exceptions that also exist in the case of PCOS patients, that even if they have a polycystic ovarian morphology, it does not mean they have PCOS. Even several studies also suggest that up to 23% of women develop PCOS without displaying any signs and symptoms, hence indicating that imaging findings are very important for timely diagnosis of the disease to avoid further complications (van der Ham et al., 2025). PCOM(polycystic ovarian morphology) is represented by a **string of pearls** sign, where numerous small antral follicles are arranged peripherally around an echogenic stroma. The subjective impressions of morphology are taken into account over the quantitative assessment of follicle number and ovarian volume, quantitative assessment is important (Di Michele et al., 2025). Among existing medical diagnostic technologies, such as CT and MRI, ultrasound is preferred primarily because of its low cost, safety, and immediate results. However, manual follicle counting is time-consuming and subjective, and it can lead to variations in reports generated by different radiologists.

b) Magnetic Resonance Imaging (MRI):

Magnetic resonance imaging is a medical imaging technique that uses a strong magnetic field and radio waves to create detailed images of the body's internal organs, tissues, and bones. A detailed assessment of ovarian stroma and follicle distribution is possible with MRI. Generally, on T2-weighted images, the central ovarian stroma typically looks hypointense, whereas peripheral cysts look hyperintense, which collectively gives the impression of a string of pearls. The appearance of this characteristic, i.e., a string of pearls, distinguishes the polycystic ovarian morphology (PCOM) associated with polycystic ovary syndrome (PCOS) from other ovarian conditions. PCOS is not routinely diagnosed with MRI because of its high cost and limited availability (van der Ham et al., 2025). In addition to PCOS testing, granulosa cell tumors, sclerosing stromal tumors, and Sertoli-Leydig cell tumors can also be excluded. When viewed on T2-weighted images, these conditions commonly show solid components that are hypointense, which can be distinguished from the cystic nature of PCOM (Lee & Rausch, 2012).

c) Computed Tomography (CT):

Ultrasound and Magnetic Resonance Imaging have better ovarian resolutions than computed tomography for detecting PCOS due to radiation risks and lack of ovarian resolution. In the course of performing another procedure, enlarged multicystic ovaries may occur as a consequence (van der Ham et al., 2022). There are multiple diagnostic tools available, but ultrasound imaging is the most common, allowing evaluations of follicle count, size, and distribution, and ovarian volume and function (Zhu et al., 2016).

1.3 TECHNICAL BACKGROUND OF POLYCYSTIC OVARY SYNDROME (PCOS)

Identifying and monitoring PCOS mainly depends on imaging and lab tests, but challenges like the skill of the operator, differences in how results are interpreted, and trouble seeing follicles in obese women, teenagers, and those who haven't had sex might require using transabdominal ultrasound, which provides lower quality images. In addition, counting follicles manually can be a time-consuming and subjective task. In order to address these challenges, AI-driven image analysis has been implemented, which enhances precision, minimizes human error, and facilitates large-scale screenings. In the automated detection of polycystic ovarian morphology (PCOM), deep learning and AI-driven image analysis are becoming increasingly valuable tools, thereby reducing radiologists' workload, improving diagnostic accuracy, and allowing early and precise detection of PCOS. (B. Zhao et al., 2025). Combining AI-driven ultrasound analysis with clinical and laboratory data improves diagnosis accuracy and speed. The use of telemedicine and remote monitoring tools also empowers women in underserved areas to manage their health conditions on their own. Additionally, telemedicine and remote monitoring tools empower women to manage their health on their own, particularly in underserved areas. Women of reproductive age are more likely to suffer from polycystic ovary syndrome (PCOS), a disorder often associated with metabolic dysfunction and insulin resistance (H. Zhao et al., 2023). An insulin sensitizing agent and an anti-androgen medication are potential treatments for PCOS. Ultrasound is the imaging modality most commonly used in the clinical evaluation of patients with ovarian illness (S. Singh et al., 2023). CT offers advantages over other medical imaging methods, such as MRI, and each has its place. The rationale is that ultrasonography is inexpensive, easily accessible, safer, and yields immediate findings for image analysis and computer vision. Deep learning is a potent technique. Early PCOS diagnosis is aided by automatic classification based on ultrasound pictures and clinical information (Hussain et al., 2022). The exploration can be more objective and diagnostically precise by employing imaging technologies to develop a deep learning model for autonomous prediction. Different criteria are used for PCOS diagnosis and symptoms that require ultrasounds, good menstrual information, and blood tests (Panjwani et al., 2025). Consequently, because this syndrome's symptoms are diverse and there is no single clinical diagnostic test or technique, medical professionals are forced to propose several clinical tests that are unnecessary for radiologic imaging. As a result, PCOS is identified by eliminating unnecessary symptoms or test findings due to the inability to comprehend the complex pathophysiological mechanism (Suha & Islam, 2023).

1.3.1 AI AND DEEP LEARNING IN PCOS DIAGNOSIS

Manual diagnosis of PCOS using ultrasound imaging and hormonal assays is inherently prone to inter-observer variability, time-consuming procedures, and limited scalability in resource-constrained settings (Christ & Cedars, 2023). In order to overcome these obstacles, we need a decision-making process that is intelligent, robust, and capable of making objective, replicable judgments. Deep learning, in particular, is crucial to addressing this problem (Amangeldy et al., 2025). Using automated data analysis, large-scale screening can be accomplished quickly, consistently, and identifies subtle patterns that are often overlooked by human evaluation, which greatly improves diagnostic accuracy. Thus, AI-based decision support systems are beneficial to PCOS patients (Khalifa & Albadawy, 2024).

a) Ultrasound image analysis: a role for deep learning

Convolutional neural networks (CNNs) are particularly effective for classifying PCOS in ovarian ultrasound images. CNNs can recognize hierarchical features in medical images and automatically perform tasks including follicle segmentation, ovary detection, and polycystic ovarian morphology (PCOM) detection (Suha & Islam, 2022). A ResNet architecture can be used here to precisely define follicular boundaries, while YOLO can be used later to detect and classify objects with high accuracy. With these models, ultrasound data can be analyzed efficiently to detect polycystic ovaries early and accurately (Neha et al., 2025).

b) Integration of Multimodal Data

To increase diagnostic precision, researchers have developed models that incorporate multimodal data, integrating clinical and laboratory factors such as body mass index(BMI), insulin levels, Anti-Mullerian hormone(AMH), and LH/FSH ratios with ultrasound image features (Le et al., 2019). This integrated approach combines conventional machine learning algorithms such as Support Vector Machines (SVMs) and Random Forest classifiers with hybrid neural networks, such as CNNs for image data and Artificial Neural Networks (ANNs) for structured clinical data. Multimodal models provide more accurate classifications than single-modality approaches because they process diverse inputs to produce a comprehensive diagnostic output (Lazri & Ameur, 2018). Below Fig. 1.6 illustrates the technological advancements of the PCOS.

c) Transfer Learning and Pre-trained Models

When analyzing medical images such as ultrasound scans, transfer learning plays a vital role in PCOS detection accuracy by leveraging pre-trained deep learning models like Inception_V3, VGG16, or MobileNet.(Lalitha & Y MD, 2024). Using this method, models can be fine-tuned after they have already been trained on a large dataset, reducing the need for large custom datasets and training from scratch. As a result, tasks like identifying PCOS-positive ovaries can be developed faster and with higher performance. In studies, these methods have also been found to be accurate enough to achieve 99.48% (J. Liu, Chui, et al., 2023).

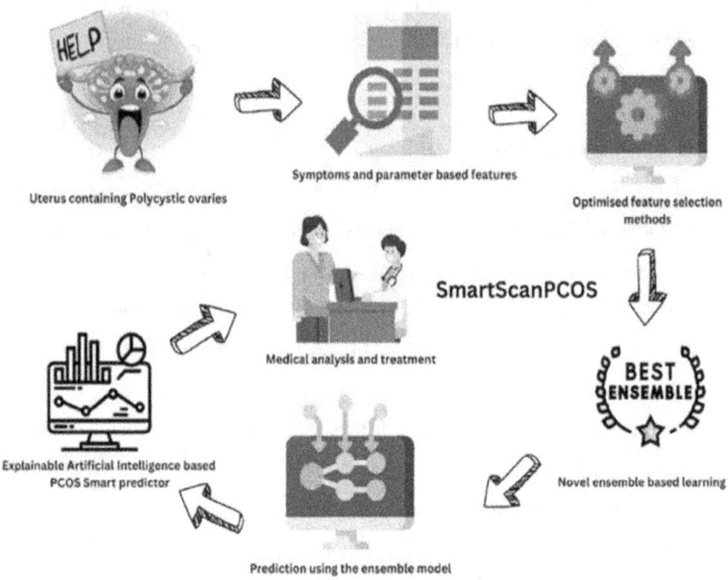

Fig. 1.6 Technological Advancements in PCOS Detection (G & P, 2024)

d) Performance evaluation metrics

Performance metrics, or parameters, are key components of the standard classification process and are used to evaluate the effectiveness of AI and deep learning models in diagnosing PCOS. In assessing the model's accuracy and balance, metrics such as accuracy, precision, recall, and F1-score are typically used and reported. Using the area under the curve (AUC) as well as receiver operating characteristics (ROC), these models are evaluated for their ability to distinguish between classes.(G & P, 2024). Based on the confusion matrix, a true positive will be compared to a false positive and vice versa; a true negative will be compared with a false negative, as well as the model's behavior will be compared. Despite many studies reporting diagnostic accuracy of over 90% under controlled experimental conditions, real-world applications across a wide range of populations and clinical settings are still crucial to the technology's development (Ahmad et al., 2024).

e) Future developments in the diagnosis of PCOS

As new technologies are integrated into PCOS diagnosis, the field is undergoing a major paradigm shift. In resource-constrained settings, AI-driven point-of-care diagnostic systems are a promising method for providing expert-level diagnosis. Portable, mobile-connected ultrasound scanners embedded with artificial intelligence may allow front-line healthcare professionals to provide high-quality diagnostic evaluations in underserved and rural areas (Verma et al., 2024). Cloud-based analytics and telemedicine platforms can significantly democratize access to PCOS treatment, especially in poor or middle-income countries with little access to specialized endocrinology care. The transformation of this complex data into actionable clinical information can be achieved through the use of deep learning models, especially those that can handle multi-omics data in high dimensions. In spite of considerable progress, AI-driven PCOS diagnostic tools remain difficult to use (J. Wang et al., 2025). In order to train and validate a robust machine learning model, large, diverse, and well-annotated datasets are required. There is a concern about generalizability and fairness of AI systems implemented across diverse populations due to the small size and lack of demographic diversity of the existing datasets. There are no standardized benchmarking techniques that make it possible to compare the results of different algorithms or studies. AI conclusions are still not explainable, and there are still concerns about patient consent, data privacy, medical liability, and medical liability for algorithmic errors (Elmannai et al., 2023b). Additionally, integration into existing healthcare workflows is hampered by technical obstacles. There are many challenges to overcome, including compatibility issues between artificial intelligence diagnostic systems, imaging equipment, and electronic health records (EHRs). Considering these limitations, it is necessary to continue investing in data infrastructure, collaborating with several institutions, and conducting longitudinal validation studies to ensure that artificial intelligence-based diagnostic solutions are both safe and effective and are also accessible to all (Nair et al., 2024).

1.4 MOTIVATION OF THE RESEARCH

Globally, nearly 116 million women have PCOS, which is a major health concern for the WHO. It is estimated that 18% of women in India suffer from the disorder, whereas approximately 5 million women in the United States are affected. It is important to raise awareness about PCOS because it affects the body beyond reproductive difficulties. As a result, you are more likely to develop breast, endometrial, or urinary cancers in the long term. PCOS is also increasingly prevalent, with about 16% of women aged 20-29 living with the condition, according to recent studies. Several studies highlight the importance of early disease diagnosis to ensure timely treatment and to prevent long-term complications. It is important to recognize that early intervention doesn't just relieve irregular cycles, hyperandrogenism, and ovarian dysfunction, but also prevents future health risks like type-2 diabetes, diabetes-related cardiovascular disease, and certain types of cancer. In order to safeguard the health and quality of life of young women around the world, it is crucial to raise awareness of the early signs of PCOS and encourage prompt medical evaluation.

1.5 RESEARCH GAP

1) Currently, collecting additional information on patients with PCOS and employing data balancing techniques has not led to a significant improvement in the dataset.

2) To determine which characteristics are optimal for classifying PCOS, no comparative analysis has been conducted.
3) Ultrasound images are affected by speckle noise, or multiplicative noise, but the majority of research has ignored this fact and instead employs additive noise filtering.
4) The majority of work is focused on follicle segmentation, while PCOS classification receives only a small amount of attention.
5) Multiple CNN architectures have been used to detect PCOS, but their accuracy has not been adequate.
6) All transfer learning techniques have not been previously employed, which allows transfer learning models to potentially be game-changing for improved results. High-resolution images, such as 3D images, will improve prediction accuracy.

1.6 RESEARCH QUESTIONS

A complex and heterogeneous disease like Polycystic Ovary Syndrome (PCOS) makes accurate early detection difficult. There are many conventional diagnostic methods that are unreliable, subjective, and resource-intensive, such as ultrasound imaging, hormonal testing, and clinical assessments. However, deep learning remains very limited in its use in PCOS diagnosis, just as it is in medical diagnostics. There are several factors that restrict the development of AI-based PCOS diagnostic systems. These include overfitting on datasets, extremely high computational demands, difficulty interpreting models, and limited generalization across populations. These gaps were filled by developing and testing improved deep learning methods for PCOS diagnosis, such as ultrasound imaging with biochemical and clinical data. Having an automated, interpretable, and clinically-translatable diagnostic paradigm will be essential for assessing PCOS accurately. We guide our study with the following questions, as discussed below:

Question 1 : Are there any existing limitations to traditional deep learning-based methods for accurately detecting PCOS from clinical, biochemical, and imaging data?

According to a variety of studies, machine learning and deep learning models perform well for image classification due to their high accuracy. Due to the small and non-diverse datasets used in most existing models, generalizability remains limited. The purpose of this study is to examine the shortcomings of these methods through a critical literature review and performance benchmarking.

Question 2: What are the best techniques for improving PCOS detection accuracy, reducing computation costs, and optimizing deep learning models?

Deep learning methods require large amounts of labeled data and computational power in real-world clinical settings, which makes their implementation difficult. Optimum strategies are used to boost performance even with limited resources and data, such as transfer learning with pretrained networks, model pruning, hyperparameter tuning, and efficient architectural designs, such as lightweight CNNs and attention mechanisms. It explores the use of these optimization techniques and assesses how they affect the accuracy, efficiency, and reproducibility of ultrasound-based PCOS detection.

Question 3: Does multimodal deep learning have the potential to improve diagnostic performance over single-input deep learning models combining ultrasound imaging, hormone profiles, and clinical symptoms?

PCOS is usually diagnosed by evaluating ultrasound imaging parameters such as ovarian volume and follicle count, as well as biochemical indicators such as LH, FSH, testosterone, and insulin levels and clinical signs such as hirsutism and irregular menstruation. It is possible to miss important diagnostic indicators when relying on one data modality only. Using a hybrid CNN-ANN or CNN-RNN model as part of the research, we examine whether better prediction, sensitivity, and specificity can be achieved when the models are integrated within a unified deep learning framework.

Question 4: In creating confidence in AI-assisted clinical diagnosis, what effect can interpretability tools, including Grad-CAM or SHAP, have on elucidating the decision-making processes made by deep learning models for PCOS detection?

In medicine, deep learning models have limitations due to their black-box nature, as clinicians may be hesitant to trust or act on recommendations without clear explanations of how they reached their conclusions. It examines ways to make deep learning models more understandable, including Gradient-weighted Class Activation Mapping (Grad-CAM) for finding images' important parts, and SHAP (SHAPley Additive exPlanations). By improving the model's transparency, building clinician trust, and ensuring AI deployment ethically, the goal is to ensure that it is deployed ethically.

Question 5: What are the characteristics of the proposed optimized deep learning model that make it suitable for deployment in real-world clinical contexts, including environments with limited resources or mobile health apps?

In order to achieve a significant clinical impact, a developed system must be scalable, exhibit minimal latency, and be compatible with a variety of operational environments. Typical scenarios include rural clinics without access to high-performance computing infrastructure or mobile diagnostic units in rural settings. This research looks at different ways to set up the system, like reducing the model size, using local processing, and cloud services, and checks how practical it is to use the improved PCOS detection model in everyday and mobile

1.7 OBJECTIVE OF THE RESEARCH

Using deep learning models for domain-specific applications such as medical image analysis, we hope to develop a model that is more efficient and accurate than existing deep learning models. Despite their power, traditional deep learning architectures have long training times, over parameterization, and limited generalization when applied to complex, high-dimensional datasets. The purpose of this study is to improve performance without compromising computational feasibility in order to overcome the drawbacks discussed above. This research aims to accomplish the following specific objectives:

(i) Evaluating the existing deep learning models like CNN, ResNet, DenseNet, and EfficientNet, using domain-specific datasets, and identifying their limitations in terms of computational complexity, convergence, and overfitting.

(ii) With the aim of enhancing performance on imbalanced datasets, an optimized deep learning architecture has been devised that combines transfer learning, batch normalization, attention mechanisms, or lightweight convolutional blocks for enhancing performance on imbalanced datasets.

(iii)In order to evaluate the high-performing deep learning model, standard metrics such as accuracy, precision, recall, F1-score, AUC-ROC, and computational efficiency were applied to real-world datasets like medical imaging and PCOS-related datasets.

(iv)In order to improve interpretability, the proposed model was then compared to baselines using a combination of quantitative and qualitative evaluation methodologies; these included tools such as Grad-CAM to improve visualization.

This research has the following scope:

a. To propose a novel method for accurate and interpretable PCOS diagnosis using ultrasound images.
b. An algorithm was developed to assist doctors, physicians, and analysts in detecting PCOS in the most optimal manner.
c. The classification of the ovary facilitates accurate diagnosis, decision-making, and further treatment, which is helpful for medical practitioners.
d. The accuracy can be obtained at the maximum possible level.

1.8 ORGANIZATION OF THESIS

Chapter 1: A general introduction to PCOS symptoms and issues, as well as the types of ovaries, the main objective, and the problem description.

Chapter 2: Explains the literature study of an overview of ovarian classification and PCOS detection, and provides the pertinent research on introductions to preprocessing, segmentation, detection, and classification techniques.

Chapter 3: Describes different materials and methodologies adopted for pre-processing, segmentation, feature extraction, and the classification process.

Chapter 4: Gives details about the results of various experimental setups for achieving all the objectives.

Chapter 5: This chapter presents the summary and findings of the overall research, as well as its connection to the Sustainable Development Goals.

1.9 CHAPTER SUMMARY

This chapter describes about what is polycystic ovary syndrome what are its characteristics and detailed signs and symptoms. A polycystic ovary syndrome patient faces a variety of challenges, as it is multifactorial and endocrine disorder that affects approximately 10-15% of women of reproductive age worldwide. This chapter also discusses about the lifelong implications of an individual's reproductive, metabolic, and psychological health. It highlights the medical urgency for an early detection of PCOS its relationship towards infertility, obesity, type 2 diabetes, cardiovascular disease, and mental health disorders such as anxiety and depression. A detailed overview of PCOS, its symptoms, hormonal imbalances, and the characteristic **"string of pearls"** appearance of polycystic ovaries seen in ultrasound imaging has been also a part of this chapter. Later the chapter talks about types of ovaries in a woman's body, namely the normal ovary, ovarian cyst, and polycystic ovary, all of which are differentiated by factors like their size, follicle count, and ultrasound characteristics. The **medical background** section of this chapter explains the hormonal disruption associated with the hypothalamic-pituitary-ovarian (HPO) axis and insulin resistance, and highlights the diagnostic difficulties when using the **Rotterdam Criteria**. Additionally, adolescents' clinical heterogeneity and similarity to normal puberty makes diagnosis more difficult. A technical background of the study highlights the disadvantages of manually interpreting ultrasound reports and laboratory tests, which supports the use of artificial intelligence (AI) and deep learning techniques to identify PCOS. Through the use of AI-powered diagnostic tools, ultrasound imaging, biochemical markers such as **LH, FSH**, testosterone, **AMH,** insulin, and clinical features can be combined to deliver better outcomes and accuracy. These scenarios can be addressed using CNNs, transfer learning, and multimodal architectures. In addition to overfitting, poor generalization, and lack of multimodal integration, the problem statement highlights the deficiencies of current deep learning models. In this way, ultrasound data, in conjunction with biochemical markers, can improve the classification of PCOS. In addition to analyzing current deep learning methods, removing noise from images, developing optimized models, evaluating using standard metrics, enhancing interpretability with Grad-CAM or SHAP, and evaluating deployment feasibility on mobile platforms, the chapter also discusses research objectives. As well as describing existing challenges and optimization strategies, multimodal integration, interpretability, and scalability, the book also outlines research questions that address these challenges.

CHAPTER 2
LITERATURE REVIEW

2.1 INTRODUCTION

In their reproductive years, women with Polycystic Ovary Syndrome (PCOS), a common endocrine disorder, suffer from the condition. PCOS must be diagnosed accurately and promptly in order to provide the best possible care and avoid related health problems. When women with PCOS have irregular periods, ultrasound images are often used to assess the development of follicles and ovarian morphology. As a result of the fact that multiple observers interpret the same images, ultrasound image interpretation is often manual and subject to subjectivity and variability. In the last few years, data analysis and algorithm development for PCOS diagnosis have progressed to the point that they can be automated and fairly objective (Reka et al., 2025). Preparing pictures is the first step in enhancing the equality and interpretability of ultrasound images, which is essential when diagnosing PCOS. It is possible to improve the accuracy of next-generation image segmentation by reducing noise, improving image quality, and normalizing images. It enables the identification and delineation of regions of interest within the ovarian stroma and follicles using ultrasound images. A high level of segmentation accuracy is required to obtain discriminative and relevant features that enable the differential diagnosis of PCOS patients from healthy controls. In feature extraction, distinguishing and relevant features are extracted from the divided regions of interest (Institutions & Krishnamoorthy, 2024). As well as textural characteristics of the ovarian stroma, morphological characteristics such as the size, shape, and distribution of the ovarian follicles could also be considered. Achieving precision in PCOS classification depends on identifying features that can help distinguish the condition from other conditions. A classification of PCOS patients based on the extracted characteristics is made, and morphological traits that are not associated with PCOS are predicted. Patients with PCOS can be classified using collected data. In order to diagnose PCOS from ultrasound images, several deep learning methods have been used, including support vector machines (SVMs), random forests (RFs), and convolutional neural networks (CNNs). In addition to the retrieved features, the performance criteria determine which classification algorithm should be selected (Elmannai et al., 2023b). The purpose of this chapter is to provide an exhaustive review of the literature related to improved deep learning methods for identifying Polycystic Ovary Syndrome (PCOS). There are four sections in this chapter. A critical evaluation of the diagnostic criteria used in recent studies is presented in Section 1 along with a discussion of the deep learning methods used in each diagnostic procedure. As part of Section 2, we present a comprehensive analysis of TV-US image preprocessing, highlighting their current limits. In Section 3, we review the current state of image segmentation, so that we can better understand its limitations and observations about ultrasound images. Section 4 examines prior research on feature extraction and classification of PCOS based on its anatomical characteristics. These three parts will elucidate the essential role of these components in improving the accuracy and reliability of PCOS diagnosis.

2.2 RESEARCH ON THE PCOS DIAGNOSTICS

While the earliest descriptions of PCOS date back to the 1930s, both diagnosis and diagnostic criteria for PCOS have evolved, and institutionalized criteria have emerged only in the past 3 decades. As more is known about PCOS, the variables that contribute to this illness also evolve, and so do the treatment and management strategies based on the profile of the individual patient. This demonstrates that PCOS symptoms are heterogenous such that treatment response to different phenotypes of the syndrome is not uniform was not until the 1990s that formal diagnostic criteria began to emerge.

The most widely referenced criteria come from the National Institutes of Health(NIH) in 1990, the Rotterdam in 2003, and the Androgen Excess Society (AES) criteria in 2006. As the understanding of PCOS has progressed, so too have the implications for treatment and management strategies tailored to individual patient profiles (Teede, Tay, Laven, Dokras, Moran, et al., 2023). A personalized approach to treatment is necessary when dealing with PCOS symptoms, as different phenotypes respond differently to treatment. Further, women with hypothyroidism may benefit from weight loss and exercise by improving insulin sensitivity and hormonal balance. In addition to addressing the immediate issues associated with PCOS, this multipronged approach aims to prevent its long-term complications, such as diabetes type 2 and vascular complications, underlining the importance of continuing research into effective PCOS treatment. The American Society for Reproductive Medicine (ASRM) recommends both metabolic and morphological analyses in recent PCOS diagnostic guidelines. The diagnostic criteria for PCOS have changed over the years. The criteria present each understanding of PCOS and reflect on what was understood before and during it, with respect to treatment and management (Sabag et al., 2024). The PCOS diagnosis is based on three important clinical parameters, such as ovulatory dysfunction and hyperandrogenism.

Ovulatory Dysfunction is the irregular or absent ovulation. It is a feature in the diagnosis of PCOS is termed oligo-anovulation. It is a feature in the diagnosis of PCOS is termed oligo-anovulation. It is an inadequate menstrual cycle, defined as more than 35 days between periods or fewer than eight periods a year. Although anovulation results in amenorrhea(absence of menstrual bleeding) in most cases, the complete non-appearance of ovulation is anovulation. Oligoanovulation, however, is a feature of women who have PCOS, which has the potential to cause reproductive dysfunction, such as infertility and increased risk of endometrial hyperplasia secondary to prolonged unopposed estrogen exposure (Lujan et al., 2008).

Hyperandrogenism is the excess of androgens (male hormones) in women, seen biochemically or clinically. Signs of hyperandrogenism can be clinical, such as hirsutism (increased hair in most areas of the body that is usually male-patterned), acne, and scalp hair thinning(overt androgenic alopecia). Laboratory tests that measure serum androgen levels, such as testosterone and DHEAS (dehydroepiandrosterone sulfate), are used to identify biochemical hyperandrogenism. Diagnosing PCOS may be clinically necessary if it is severe (Yildiz, 2006).

Polycystic Ovary Morphology (PCOM) is characterized by multiple small follicles (cysts) on the ovarian walls, which can be visualized on ultrasound. According to Rotterdam, PCOS diagnosis can include multiple cysts in the ovaries, characterised by 12 or more follicles measuring 2-9mm in diameter in one or both ovaries, along with an increased ovarian volume (more than 10 cm^3). (Rotterdam ESHRE/ASRM-Sponsored) PCOS Consensus workshop group,2004). The presence of PCOM is significant as it reflects the underlying hormonal imbalance and disrupted ovarian function associated with PCOS (Lujan et al., 2008).

2.3 IMAGE PRE-PROCESSING

Image preprocessing serves as a foundational step in computer-aided diagnostic systems, ensuring that medical images are prepared for reliable analysis and interpretation. It is imperative that preprocessing is performed prior to ultrasound-based detection of polycystic ovary syndrome (PCOS) due to the inherent challenges of ultrasound imaging, such as low contrast, shadowing, intensity inhomogeneity, and speckle noise (J. Liu, Li, et al., 2023). Through preprocessing, input data is improved in clarity and uniformity while clinically relevant structures are preserved, improving the performance of subsequent segmentation, feature extraction, and classification. Among the standard preprocessing operations are normalization and contrast enhancement, which enhance the visibility of ovarian morphology and follicular boundaries; histogram equalization and adaptive contrast methods, which highlight subtle textural variations; and geometric transformations to standardize the dataset and increase model generalization. During the preprocessing of deep learning pipelines, data augmentation techniques like flipping, scaling, and brightness variation are used to enhance data saturation and reduce overfitting, helping to ensure robust performance of deep learning models across a wide range of patient populations (Salvi et al., 2021). The accuracy of diagnostic imaging depends heavily on the reduction of noise in ultrasound images when they are being preprocessed, since speckle noise generally obscures fine details. Most traditional denoising methods, including median and Wiener filters, anisotropic diffusion, and wavelet-based thresholding, are limited in their ability to reduce noise while maintaining anatomical details. There are a number of features that are necessary to diagnose PCOS, such as peripheral follicular arrangement, increased ovarian volume, and hyperechogenic stroma. In this regard, maintaining structural fidelity is essential(J. Liu, Li, et al., 2023). With recent advances in deep learning, more sophisticated denoising solutions have been developed, including convolutional neural networks (CNNs), autoencoders, and generative adversarial networks (GANs), which learn directly from training data the characteristics of noise and structural priors. The effectiveness of these models is demonstrated by the fact that they effectively suppress speckle noise while retaining the edge and texture information crucial for ovarian assessment (Nazir et al., 2024). It is also possible to enhance noise reduction effectiveness by implementing optimized strategies-such as task-specific training on ovarian ultrasound datasets, multiobjective optimization that maximizes structural similarity and diagnostic accuracy, and transfer learning from larger ultrasound repositories. A combination of preprocessing and denoising steps can improve the accuracy of automated PCOS detection systems when incorporated into deep learning frameworks (Shanmugavadivel et al., 2024). In this thesis, a comprehensive approach to image pre-processing has been developed to deliver ultrasound images that are effectively denoised. Following are the steps taken to achieve this goal:

i. **Standardization of dimensions:** The images are all resized to 128x128x3. As a result of this standardization, the input data always maintains uniform dimensions, which is necessary for the deep learning model to be able to effectively process the images.

ii. **Normalization:** It is necessary to normalize the pixels in order to bring them within a certain range. The process ensures that all images are of comparable intensity, which stabilizes and speeds up the training process.

iii. **Smoothing:** Using image smoothing techniques, small artifacts are reduced while critical features are maintained. In this step, the image quality is enhanced and irrelevant details are removed that might interfere with the denoising process.

iv. **Synthetic Noise Addition:** Speckle noise at different variance levels (0.001, 0.02, and 0.5) is artificially added to the images to simulate real-world conditions. By enhancing the model with this feature, it becomes able to denoise images more effectively with varying noise intensities, increasing its robustness.

By performing these pre-processing operations, we are ensuring that the dataset we create will be consistent, clean, and representative of ultrasound imaging scenarios that we encounter in practice. Their main advantage is that they facilitate more accurate feature extraction by the autoencoder's attention mechanism, ultimately improving denoising performance and diagnostic utility.

In terms of background research, these are the major studies:

Denny et al. (Denny et al., 2019) applied machine learning to create i-HOPE, which detects and predicts Polycystic Ovary Syndrome (PCOS). There were 541 females with PCOS in the study, aged 18-40, with 177 cases. A number of factors are evaluated, including accuracy, precision, sensitivity/recall, specificity, and the F1 score. According to the research, Random Forest Classifier (RFC) performed better than other machine learning algorithms. In this case, a holdout validation set is used in testing the data and optimizing the model.

Bharati et al. (Bharati et al., 2022) explained data-driven PCOS diagnosis. He evaluated an ensemble machine learning algorithm on training data from Kaggle. The dataset comprises 43 characteristics of 177 PCOS-positive women. A univariate feature selection and feature exclusion technique is used to determine the best PCOS predictors. Most essential is the FSH/LH ratio. Dataset classifiers include voting hard, voting soft, and CatBoost.

Mehr et al. (Rahman et al., 2024) described that machine learning techniques and feature selection approaches are used to diagnose polycystic ovarian syndrome (PCOS). Several types of patterns were used in the analysis of the Kaggle PCOS clinical dataset, including a Multi-Layer Perceptron, an Ensemble Random Forest, an Ensemble Boosting, and an Ensemble Extra Tree. Additionally, they assessed the accuracy of each classifier after varying the strategies for selecting features. A review of machine learning techniques and feature selection has been conducted to diagnose PCOS in this report. In their study, the authors briefly describe the classification algorithms, feature selection methodologies, and dataset used for the study. The study discusses the techniques used for categorizing and selecting features, as well as the findings and conclusions of the experiment.

Alamoudi et al. (Alamoudi et al., 2023) proposed a deep learning fusion approach in order to detect Polycystic Ovary Syndrome (PCOS), a hormonal disorder afflicting women of reproductive age, and one of the most significant causes of infertility among women. PCOS is diagnosed by Rotterdam criteria-high androgen hormones, ovulation failure as well as ultrasonography of polycystic ovaries (PCOM). The report contains ultrasound images of the ovary and clinical statistics of the PCOS and non-PCOS patients. The Inception model was able to diagnose PCOM using the ultrasound image with the 84.81% accuracy.

By **Sheela et al.** (S, V, et al., 2020) the ultrasonography segmentation techniques of ovarian cysts were compared Accurate segmentation is the key in the analysis of polycystic ovarian images as they may differ between patients, which is pointed out by the authors. The paper has been comparing performance of various segmentation algorithms, which include Level set algorithm, Adaptive thresholding, and K-means clustering, based on parameters of performance matrices. The authors conclude that adaptive thresholding technique is the best when it comes to a more precise division of ovarian cysts in ultrasound images.

Yusof et al. (Hiremath & Tegnoor, 2010) proposed a computational model aimed at determining and estimating the number of and the diameter of ovarian follicles in ultrasound images by using machine learning. The model combines preprocessing, segmentation, speckle amplification, attenuation of noises of follicles, feature extraction and selection, and calculation of the follicular diameters to determine the number of follicles. This segmentation is done through an active-contour algorithm, which uses morphological similarities between the follicles, and thus, this algorithm offers the ability to accurately determine the number and diameter of the follicles. The success of the method is evaluated by means of Probabilistic Rand Index (PRI) and Global Consistency Error (GCE) measures on data consisting of patient ovarian ultrasound images.

Vinodhini et al. (Jeyalakshmi & Ramar, 2010) aimed at using changed wavelet filters in images of an ultrasonic scan of polycystic ovary syndrome (PCOS). The importance of medical images preprocessing to remove speckle noise is highlighted in the study because it otherwise reduces the quality of the ultrasound and computed-tomography scans. The authors conclude that the proposed filter works well in cyst detection of ultrasound images of PCOS, where the peak signal-to-noise ratio (PSNR), signal-to-noise ratio (SNR), and structural similarity index (SSIM) are used as a measure of performance across all types of discrete wavelet transforms.

Jeevitha et al. (Jeevitha & Priya, 2022a) suggested a new SCBOD approach to the recognition of PCOS basing on the classification of the follicles and the ovary. Its methodology is based on four steps, namely preprocessing, segmentation, SCBOD detection, and SVM classification.

Nazarudin et al. (Nazarudin et al., 2020) investigated the diagnosis of polycystic ovarian syndrome (PCOS) by ultrasound imaging that is a non-invasive and time-saving modality. The treatment of PCOS requires the accurate determination of ovarian follicles. Manually identifying follicles is time-consuming and error-prone. Researchers have investigated automated follicle identification methods. The study reviews prior image segmentation methods and algorithms for automated follicle identification in PCOS diagnosis. The publication also proposes research approaches.

He et al. (Elmannai et al., 2023b) offered a learnt image quality kernel probabilistic model for identifying Polycystic Ovary Syndrome (PCOS). The model represents each picture as a score matrix and generates a long feature vector from grayscale and texture features. A probabilistic model learns this feature vector and feeds it into an SVM kernel for PCOS identification. The proposed PCOS detection technique works. Image quality diagnosis technology can identify endometrial thickness and changes in ovarian blood flow speed and resistance in PCOS patients, helping with disease diagnosis and treatment prognosis.

Gopalakrishnan et al. (Suha & Islam, 2022) addressed the endocrine disorder polycystic ovary syndrome (PCOS), which affects 5-10% of women of reproductive age. Infertility is a clinical, endocrinological, and biochemical manifestation of abnormalities in the estrogen and androgen metabolism in women with PCOS. Most immature follicles, those smaller than 10 mm in diameter, are found at the ovaries' perimeter. Ultrasound pictures are now used to help clinicians detect and analyze PCOS by identifying the number, size, and location of follicles. However, due to variations in follicle size and their linkages to tissues and blood vessels, real-time analysis of follicles is prone to mistakes.

Pradeepa et al. (Pradeepa et al., 2023) developed a methodology named DEODORANT, a unique association rule-based hypergraph model for early detection and prevention of PCOS. NLTK preprocesses unstructured media input, and the apriori algorithm derives association rules. To form clusters, these hypergraph association rules are regenerated as line graphs. Spectral clustering divides the line graph into hypergraph groups. The required conclusions about the hypergraph can be drawn by applying the dominating set property. The data show that the experimentally determined outcome supports values, ranked by percentage. This research will help medical professionals track patients' symptoms and illnesses, enabling early diagnosis and successful treatment.

Mandal et al. (Mandal et al., 2021) used K-means clustering to automatically segment ovarian ultrasound follicles. Ovarian follicle quantity, shape, and size can help diagnose and monitor disorders such as infertility, PCOS, ovarian cancer, and others. The suggested technique divided follicles out of nineteen ultrasound images. The paper also describes loading ultrasound images, computing their histograms, equalizing, reshaping the data to a two-dimensional array, K-means clustering and morphological erosion to come up with the final segmented image.

Choubey et al. (Choubey et al., 2021) developed a two-step image denoising algorithm used to identify polycystic ovarian syndrome (PCOS) using transvaginal an ultrasound image. An image's noise properties are identified in the first stage, and then specific filters are applied to generate a noise-free image in the second stage. In comparison with existing methods, this paper reports a significant reduction in Mean Squared Error (MSE) for salt-and-pepper, Gaussian, and speckle noise. PCOS should be detected and treated early, as highlighted in the paper, with the use of advanced imaging techniques.

Acharya et al. (Acharya et al., 2013) discussed the clinical and nonclinical criteria used to distinguish benign from malignant ovarian tumors. In addition, the report discusses the development of CAD systems that automatically distinguish benign from malignant ovarian tumors. In ultrasound-based CAD systems, classifiers are critical. This paper summarizes the characteristics of ovarian tissue using ultrasonography.

Gopalakrishnan et al. (Gopalakrishnan & Iyapparaja, 2020) suggested by method for diagnosing Polycystic Ovary Syndrome (PCOS) from ovarian ultrasound pictures. A modified Otsu threshold is used to detect the number and size of ovarian follicles using an active contour. The difficulty of assessing follicular size and connection to blood vessels and tissues makes PCOS difficult to diagnose. The suggested method selects the best filter from a set of conventional filters before preprocessing the ovary picture. According to the research, the proposed segmentation algorithm performs better than the others.

Sheela et al. (S, M, et al., 2020) discussed the difficulties of evaluating ultrasound pictures to diagnose polycystic ovarian syndrome (PCOS), a leading cause of female infertility. Researchers present a technique for segmenting ultrasound ROIs that works well with all image types, called Adaptive Otsu's Technique (AOT). Also discussed in the study are the pros and cons of ultrasound imaging for diagnosing PCOS, including image quality, noise, follicle overlap, and inexperienced operators. AOT segmented ultrasonic ROIs more effectively than conventional methods, according to the article.

Deng et al. (Deng et al., 2011) provided a system of ultrasound-based automated diagnosis of PCOS. The two key functional components of the system include the preprocessing phase and follicle identification due to the growth of objects. We evaluated the accuracy of the proposed approach against three known methods on 31 real PCOS ultrasound images that were taken on patients. The BVF method, the level set technique and the FSVM classifier are applied to diagnose RR and MR values.

Suha et al. (Suha & Islam, 2022) proposed an expanded machine learning approach Diagnosis of PCOS is best done through ovarian ultrasound scans which could reveal many cysts and this is a common endocrinological disorder that afflicts women everywhere in the world. The suggested method uses a CNN to extract features from photos and then stacks ensemble machine learning models to distinguish ovaries with and without PCOS. Compared with other machine learning-based approaches, the method improves accuracy while shortening training time. The pre-trained VGGNet16 model, combined with a CNN architecture as a feature extractor and a stacking ensemble with XGBoost as the meta-learner, yields the best results, achieving 99.89% accuracy on image classification.

Dewailly et al. (Dewailly et al., 2011) discussed the diagnosis of PCOS and the use of ultrasonography to identify polycystic ovarian morphology (PCOM). FNPO is 25, and OV is 10 ml. The article also suggests using anti-Mullerian hormone (AMH) as a surrogate marker for PCOM, although AMH testing must first be standardized. In the absence of additional PCOS symptoms, PCOM does not have substantial health repercussions, although further study is needed to completely understand its effects.

Suha et al. (Alam Suha & Islam, 2023) examined a data-driven PCOS diagnosis in women. Kaggle data trained ensemble machine learning algorithms. The collection comprises 177 PCOS women and 43 features. The authors found the best PCOS predictors using univariate feature selection and elimination. The most important ratio was FSH/LH. Feature selection and deletion used cross-validation. The dataset uses voting hard, voting soft, and CatBoost classifiers. The top 13 risk factors accurately predict the onset of PCOS.

Chen et al. (L. Chen et al., 2023) presented a new framework called Mask-guided Generative Adversarial Network (MGGAN). Artificially identified symbols that may alter the precision of lesion classification and segmentation can be found in the clinically processed 2D ovarian-tumor ultrasound images. To make lesion borders more realistic, the MGGAN uses painting-in-the-picture methods to remove symbols from images and an attention mechanism to focus on valid information while ignoring symbols. The approach improves the accuracy of computerized ovarian tumor identification and enables pixel-level painting of distorted areas in unclear images.

Maheshwari et al. (G & P, 2024) offered a new method for feature selection named Furious Flies for the classification and prediction of Polycystic Ovary Syndrome (PCOS). Adaptive histogram equalization is used in the proposed method to remove noise from photos, followed by the extraction of PCOS-related characteristics, feature selection using the Furious Flies algorithm, and image classification using artificial neural networks and a Naive Bayesian classifier. With 100% precision, an F-measure of 68.76%, and a recall of 55%, the suggested model achieves an accuracy of 98.63%.

Guha et al. (Guha & Kodipalli, 2025) used machine learning and image processing to identify and differentiate between ovarian cysts and PCOS in ultrasound images. PCOS women are usually infertile and obese, experience diabetes, and suffer a heart disease. Medical analysts and doctors find it difficult to trace and quantify ovarian follicles and this may result to inaccuracies. The way researchers ovarian categorize and detect PCOS, their characteristics, and metrics are addressed. According to the article, ultrasonic imaging involves no harm or risk, is effective in identifying gynecological disorders and processing of images can identify follicles in ovarian images depending on size and follicle count.

Zhang et al. (X. Zhang et al., 2021) described the way Raman spectroscopy with the models of principal component analysis and spectrum classification enabled them to determine the metabolic pathways in follicular fluid and plasma samples of women with PCOS. 50 healthy (non-PCOS) and 50 PCOS women provided follicular fluid and plasma samples to the study, which were analyzed using the Raman spectroscopy. The results showed that PCOS could modify metabolic states which would be observed using Raman spectroscopy. Machine learning algorithms based on Raman would classify the two groups using follicular fluid with much accuracy compared to using plasma samples. In the studies, Raman spectroscopy and sophisticated machine-learning algorithms can be used to recognize PCOS patients. To determine the metabolic patterns of follicular fluid and plasma samples of women with Polycystic Ovary Syndrome (PCOS), Raman spectroscopy, multivariate statistical techniques, and machine-learning algorithms. Principal component analysis and spectral classification models were used to analyze follicular fluid and plasma samples of 50 healthy (non-PCOS) and 50 PCOS women.

The model introduced by **Sumathi et al.** (Sumathi et al., 2021) was effective and utilized CNN-based image processing. It employs the feature extraction of the images that have undergone a CNN to classify cysts in the dataset. The proposed system is able to detect cysts in the dataset using ultrasound pictures as training data. It can then classify test data using these images as a reference to ascertain whether the ovary is affected and the specific metrics that are affected as a result, that is, its size, firmness, extension and perimeter. The independently trained dataset of the study is the same PCOS-related disorders. The article addresses the effectiveness of the proposed technique, in which the test data set is applied, and the process of the feature extraction is carried out, and the results reach 85% accuracy. Preprocessing, segmentation, and feature extraction needed in the classification, morphological operations like erosion, dilation, and others are also discussed in the study.

Purnama et al. suggested a method of determining follicles in the Ultrasound (USG) images to diagnose Polycystic Ovary Syndrome (PCOS). Using C=40 with RBF (SVM

Kernel), the proposed technique of diagnosing Polycystic Ovary Syndrome (PCOS) through identifying follicles by use of Ultrasonography (USG) images achieved an accuracy rate of 82.55% in dataset A. In the case of dataset B, KNN prevented with a classification of Euclidean distance (K=5) and reached an accuracy of 78.81%.

Nsugbe et.al. (Nsugbe, 2023) proposed AI-based decision support system of PCOS early detection. The study uses the Kaggle PCOS dataset to create a predictive model that identifies whether PCOS exists or not and the level of its severity. The model uses high-order SVM with a nonlinear boundary to deal with data that has high levels of overlap. The study also derives statistical features of the medical information to complement the feature vector obtained by utilizing the medical record of the patient, and enhance data class Separability. One of the issues that the SMOTE synthetic sample generator handles is an imbalanced sample set. The proposed plan could offer a clinical decision support tool that would facilitate an increased rate of the diagnosis and improved treatment of PCOS patients.

Karia et al. (Karia et al., 2023) created an approach named BeRedy to support menstruators in their cycle related issues. It tracks the menstrual periods, offers details of PCOD/PCOS, suggested exercises and diet, support groups and help materials and allows people to purchase menstrual supplies through reliable means. The study also addresses briefly on the gradient boosting procedure such as loss function and base-learner model to be used. Talks about menstruating people and how they would need to find a solution to assist them in managing their menstrual wellbeing. The authors suggest a program known as BeRedy that would be able to provide a variety of tools to monitor the menstrual periods, inform and empower with piece of information, prescribe exercises and alterations in the diet concerning PCOS/PCOD, find support groups, and allow buying menstrual items on reliable websites. A chatbot provides support and specific advice to individual questions concerning menstruation. The research also describes the steps of the period cycle tracker such as creating decision trees of each sample, finding the number of days between periods and average cycle length that will be used to predict the date of the next period.

A competitive neural network was deployed to classify ultrasound images of the polycystic ovary by **Dewi et al.** (Dewi et al., 2018) The authors introduce one of the approaches to diagnosing polycystic ovarian syndrome, which may lead to infertility in females. Competitive neural network is used to classify ovarian ultrasound images according to polycystic or non-polycystic.

Chitra et al. (Chitra et al., 2023) suggested the use of deep learning-based hybrid models in identifying ultrasound PCOS images. Transfer learning is used to enhance the accuracy through the combination of VGG16, AlexNet, inception V3. The improvement of results is conducted by data augmentation prior to the training of an ensemble model. The paper focuses on features selection and over-parameterization shortcomings. The PCOS image classifiers are evaluated using validation accuracy, validation loss, recall, precision and F-score.

Barber et al. (Barber et al., 2019) observed Obesity and polycystic ovarian syndrome (PCOS), a prevalent endocrinopathy affecting 6-10% of reproductive-age women, are linked. Hyperandrogenism, reproductive, metabolic, and insulin resistance define PCOS. Weight gain and obesity affect PCOS etiology, with the insulin route being the main mediator. They also evaluate food and exercise changes for obese and overweight individuals with PCOS.

Hassan et al. (Mubasher Hassan & Mirza, 2020) compared machine learning techniques for PCOS detection. His work diagnoses PCOS using clinical data and machine learning methods, including SVM, CART, Random Forest, Naïve Bayes Classification, and Logistic Regression. The random forest algorithm diagnoses PCOS with 96% accuracy.

Chauhan et al. (Chauhan et al., 2021) suggested using machine learning to predict PCOS early. PCOS, a common endocrine disorder in childbearing women, causes infertility and other problems. Python and Google Colab-cleaned survey data powers the proposed app. The essay compares KNN, Naive Bayes, Decision Tree Classifier, SVM, and LR for PCOS classification. The accuracy and confusion matrices showed that the Decision Tree Classifier performed best at predicting PCOS.

Lv et al. (Lv et al., 2022) presented an automated deep learning approach to diagnose PCOS using scleral pictures. An upgraded U-Net segments scleral pictures from full-eye images, and a ResNet model extracts features. A multi-instance model addresses many instances. The program analyzes 721 Chinese women, 388 of whom have PCOS. AUC, accuracy, recall, precision, and F1-score measure algorithm performance. The suggested method's average AUC of 0.979 and accuracy of 0.929 demonstrate the promise of deep learning for PCOS detection using scleral images.

Bharati et al. (Rahman et al., 2024) employed Polycystic ovary syndrome (PCOS) in women using machine learning algorithms. He employed a univariate feature selection method to determine that the FSH/LH ratio is the single most important predictor of PCOS. They employed holdout and cross-validation strategies, using classifiers including gradient boosting, random forest, logistic regression, and a hybrid random forest-logistic regression (RFLR) to split the data into training and test sets. Using 40-fold cross-validation on the 10 most important features, RFLR achieves 91.01% accuracy and 90% recall.

Zigarelli et al. (Zigarelli et al., 2022) identified machine learning-based self-diagnostic prediction models of polycystic ovarian syndrome (PCOS) based on non-invasive measurements including anthropometric measures, symptoms, age, and lifestyle variables. The accuracy of the patient models of predicting somebody with PCOS was 81% to 82.5% with the sole use of non-invasive measurements, whereas the provider models predicted PCOS status with an accuracy of 87.5% . Table 2.1 provides a brief summary of how machine learning and deep learning can be used to diagnose PCOS in new manners.

Table 2.1: Summary of recent machine learning and deep learning approaches for PCOS diagnosis

Author/Year	**Objective**	**Proposed Methodology**	**Results**	**Limitations**

Sumathi et al.(Wiweko & Beelonie, n.d.),2021	Automate PCOS detection from ultrasound images	Transfer learning CNNs (AlexNet, Inception V3, Resnet50,VGG 16)hybridVGG16+Resnet50;data augmentation	Acc=95% Precision=91% Sensitivity=100% Specificity=90% F1 Score=95%	Imbalanced data challenge; need precise ultrasound angle; ensembles are costly and complex
Castelino et al.(Castelino, 2023),2023	Early PCOS detection	Transfer learning using VGG-16 and Inception-V3 on ultrasound images	Acc=100% Precision=100% Recall=100%	Small, unbalanced dataset; lacks clinical details; pretrained weights not ultrasound-specific
Shanmugavadivel et al.,2024(Shanmugavadivel et al., 2024)	Early and accurate diagnosis of PCOS using clinical and ultrasound data	Machine learning (LR, NB, SVM) on clinical features; CNN and VGG16 transfer learning on ultrasound images	Acc=94.44% Precision=0.9143 Recall =0.9143	Limited by dataset size and lack of clinical validation
Ravishankar et al., 2023(Ravishankar et al., 2023)	Early detection and classification of ovarian cysts using ultrasound images	Fuzzy rule-based Convolutional Neural Network (OCD-FCNN) combining CNN feature extraction with fuzzy logic for classification	Acc=98.37%	Limited dataset size (320 training, 120 testing images); plans to increase images in future work to improve accuracy and efficiency

Rachana et al.,2021(Rachana et al., 2021a)	Early PCOS detection	Ultrasound image preprocessing, Otsu segmentation, feature extraction, KNN classification	Acc=97.43%	High KNN computational time; future optimization needed
Purnama et al.(Purnama et al., 2015), 2024	AI-based PCOS detection from ultrasound images	Preprocessing, Gabor wavelet feature extraction, classification with LVQ, KNN, SVM	Acc= 82.55%	Small dataset; some segmentation errors; feature selection needs improvement
Moral et al. 2024(Moral, Mustafi, Mustafi, et al., 2024b)	To develop an AI-driven automated system for PCOS detection and classification using ultrasound images.	Preprocessing of US images, Feature extraction using CystNet hybrid model, Classification via fully connected layers with 5-fold cross-validation and ensemble machine learning classifiers	Acc=97.75% Precision=96.23% Recall=98.29% F1-Score=97.19% Specificity=97.37%	The CystNet model is less generalizable and resilient in varied clinical contexts due to a single dataset.
Maheshwari et al,2024(Maheswari, 2025)	Accurately detect PCOS from	Hybrid model combining InceptionV3 for feature extraction and	Acc=99.3% Precision=99.2% Recall=99.3%	Dataset size limited; needs multi-modal

	ultrasound images	XGBoost for classification with image augmentation	F1 Score=99.2%	data integration.
Jeevitha & Priya,2022(Jeevitha & Priya, 2022b)	Identify and classify ovarian cysts in ultrasound images	SCBOD algorithm: preprocessing, improved watershed segmentation, size and count-based detection, SVM classification	Acc=94% Precision=100 % Recall(sensitivity)=95% F-measure=97.4 % TP Rate =95%	Difficulty distinguishing normal cysts from other cyst types; limited dataset size affecting classification accuracy
Danaei Mehr & Polat,2022(Danaei Mehr & Polat, 2022)	Diagnose PCOS using machine learning on a clinical dataset	Applied Ensemble AdaBoost, Ensemble Extra Tree, Ensemble Random Forest (RF), MLP classifiers; used feature selection (Pearson filter, RF embedded, SBS wrapper)	Acc=98.89% Sensitivity=100 %	Results based on a specific dataset; feature selection methods may risk ignoring critical features; applicability to other datasets is uncertain
Alamoudi et al., 2023(Alamoudi et al., 2023)	Develop a CAD model to diagnose PCOS using ultrasound images and clinical data	Used deep learning models (CNN architectures like Inception, MobileNet) and fusion of ultrasound image features	Acc=82.46% Precision=69.57% F1-Score=72.73% Recall=76.19%	Dataset limited to 391 images; manual labelling by radiologists; model performance dependent on the quality of

		with clinical data features for diagnosis		clinical data and images
Abouhawwash et al.(Abouhawwash et al., 2023), 2023	Improve automatic PCOS diagnosis using deep learning and feature selection	Tri-stage wrapper feature selection + DL classifiers (CNN, MLP, RNN, Bi-LSTM) on 541-subject dataset	Acc=98.67% Precision=97% Recall =89%	Weaker recall in some models; dataset regional; ultrasound image noise

Daescu et al. (Daescu et al., 2023) analyzed somatic complaints and other clinical events occurring in PCOS in relation to hyperandrogenism. The research showed that patients with BMI of 25 years and above are vulnerable to health issues. The BESAQ scale was used to define PCOS women with sexual dysfunction. Sexual dysfunction is highly predicted by the scale score, FT value, LH/FSH ratio, and the BMI. The analysis concluded that the BESAQ scale may be used by physicians to determine individuals at risk of sexual dysfunction and give them suitable intervention.

In their article, **Xie et al. (Xie et al., 2020)** presented the results of the creation and analysis of a metabolic diagnostic model of Polycystic Ovary Syndrome (PCOS) based on a random forest and an artificial neural network. The aim of the study is to identify gene biomarkers and come up with a model of PCOS diagnosis. The gene expression was found in the Gene Expression Omnibus (GEO) database and analyzed by the machine learning techniques. This paper finds that the diagnostic model is better than existing marker genes in microarray data classification and prediction.

Nusinovici et al. (Nusinovici et al., 2020) investigated the accuracy of logistic regression and machine learning in major chronic illnesses prediction with fundamental clinical variables. During the predictions, the research found out that logistic regression was equally effective as machine learning. The authors are of the opinion that this finding would be useful to healthcare providers who might not have access to the latest technology. This study assesses the effectiveness of machine learning algorithms and compares them with logistic regression in the prediction of the risk of major chronic diseases, such as cardiovascular disease, diabetes, kidney disease, and hypertension. This was a population-based cohort study on Asian adults. The authors discovered that logistic regression is equally predictive to machine learning models in estimating the risk of major chronic diseases with low incidence and easy clinical predictors. Machine learning might not be superior to regression in the prediction of low-incidence diseases.

Shami et al. (Shami et al., 2022) carried out an extensive literature review of Particle Swarm Optimization (PSO), which is a popular optimization algorithm based on the social behavior of birds and fish. The paper addresses several subjects of PSO such as its history, variants, uses, and research directions of the future. The authors also touch upon the strengths and weaknesses of different variants of PSO and provide suggestions on how to improve their work. Eight potential PSO optimization research topics are included in the report.

Nazarudin et al.(Nazarudin et al., 2023) suggested a hybrid segmentation approach for ultrasound-based PCOS diagnosis and monitoring. Otsu's thresholding and Chan-Vese segment and identify ovarian follicles. The paper compares the suggested technique to Chan-Vese in terms of accuracy, Dice score, Jaccard index, and sensitivity. The suggested technique beats Chan-Vese in sensitivity, Dice score, and Jaccard index. Otsu's thresholding and the Chan-Vese approach improve ultrasound picture segmentation for PCOS diagnosis and monitoring.

Elmannai et al. (Elmannai et al., 2023b) suggested a machine learning approach. An explainable, feature-selection-based artificial intelligence is used in the model to ensure its efficacy. The research used a variety of machine learning models, including k-nearest neighbors, logistic regression, random forests, decision trees, naive Bayes, support vector machines, and the AdaBoost algorithm, to identify the best model and the most effective feature selection. The model's explainability is examined and compared with earlier investigations. Stacking ML with RFE had the best accuracy, precision, recall, F1, and AUC, according to the experimental data. According to the study's findings, early and accurate PCOS diagnosis will aid healthcare systems in minimizing the consequences and issues associated with the condition.

The study by **Shan et al.** (Shan et al., 2015) identified the risk factors of PCOS among the Li inhabitants of China. In the case-control study, 285 PCOS were used and 580 non-PCOS cases were used. The PCOS risk factors of the Li population were menstrual cycle abnormality, low mood, family history of diabetes and infertility, mother menstrual irregularity, and physical inactivity. Early screening, diagnosis, and treatment are recommended in the research to decrease incidences of PCOS and enhance the outcomes. The paper also reveals the impact of lifestyle factors, including poor eating habits and lack of physical activities on the PCOS rates of Li.

A hybrid framework recommended by **Kumari et al.** (Kumari et al., 2023) is the so-called SmS, to be used in the early diagnosis of PCOS among women. The proposed model uses both ensemble method of stacking and oversampling method of SMOTE to enhance diagnostic accuracy. The model uses the six classifiers as base learners and it tests each of the classifiers separately at the meta-level. Another aspect of the study is the evaluation of the Logistic Regression (LR) method and the calculation of the entropy at each iteration of the algorithms. The last decision boundary is calculated based on numeric parameters acquired by means of Support Vector machine optimization. Good treatment of PCOS depends on the early diagnosis of this condition because it can cause multiple health-related problems, including diabetes type 2 and heart diseases.

Hart et al. (Hart & Doherty, 2015) emphasized research on the potential outcomes of the diagnosis of PCOS on the future health of a woman. The study indicated that women with PCOS had higher rates of hospitalization due to different health conditions, such as reproductive, metabolic, and cardiovascular diseases. PCOS women were also more likely to have diabetes and cancer. The study highlights the importance of early diagnosis and treatment of PCOS to avoid the long-term effects on the health of individuals.

2.4 CHAPTER SUMMARY

The chapter makes a thorough review of available literature about active application of optimized deep learning methods to detect and treat Polycystic Ovary Syndrome (PCOS). The chapter starts with the contextualization of the clinical framework of the PCOS and its diagnostic development by presenting the shift towards the AI-based tools that replace the traditional approach to diagnosis. It talks about the Rotterdam criteria, imaging, including ultrasound and MRI, and the importance of clinical assessment in proper diagnosis.

After that, the chapter discusses how artificial intelligence (AI) can be used in healthcare, focus on ethical considerations, explainability requirement, and the significance of interdisciplinary collaboration. It also details the growing presence of telemedicine and mobile health solutions in the PCOS care.

Much of this is focused on deep learning algorithms, such as Convolutional Neural Networks (CNNs), Recurrent Neural Networks (RNNs), Autoencoders, Transfer Learning, GANs, and Explainable AI (XAI). These are considered in terms of their usefulness in medical imaging and PCOS diagnosis, with the emphasis laid on enhancing accuracy, the strength of the model, and the efficiency of data. The models of segmentation like U-Net and Mask R-CNN are also reviewed with regards to their capability of identifying ovarian cysts.

The chapter reports the findings of many other studies that used machine learning and image processing to diagnose PCOS and the models obtained high accuracy rates with either ensemble learning, transfer learning or multimodal data fusion. It observes the need to overcome limitations which include data sparsity, extrapolation and decipherability of deep learning models.

Lastly, it also outlines gaps in research that are critical such as the necessity to include various and extensive datasets; the incorporation of individualized data (genetics and lifestyle factors); and the incorporation of community-based and digital interventions to enhance equitable healthcare access. The chapter ends by highlighting the possibility of using AI, nanotechnology and taking a holistic approach to enhance early diagnosis, a tailored treatment and long-term health outcomes in women with PCOS.

CHAPTER-3

THEORETICAL BACKGROUND AND DEEP LEARNING TECHNIQUES

3.1 INTRODUCTION

3.1.1 Overview of Deep Learning in Medical Imaging

Deep learning is a subset of artificial intelligence that has changed how machines learn, interpret, and work with large, complex datasets. The working mechanism of deep learning technology is absolutely similar to that of the neural networks in the human brain. Given the large volume of unstructured data, deep learning enables computers to find patterns and make smart decisions on their own. In modern medical imaging, deep learning has become one of the most revolutionary technologies, enabling computers to learn patterns automatically. Natural patterns are more complex than those in medical data, without the need for manually designed features (Taye, 2023). Deep learning models-especially Convolutional Neural Networks (CNNs)-are capable of fetching hierarchical, multi-level features directly from pixel data, making them highly reliable and suitable for analyzing heterogeneous and noisy medical images such as ultrasound scans in contrast to classical image-processing methodologies, which rely mainly on handcrafted descriptors. Deep learning plays a pivotal role because of the inherent inconsistencies of the modality. The problem in ultrasound scans is related to their quality because generally these images remain affected by irregularities like speckle noise, shadow artifacts, low contrast, and operator dependency, which hinder the clear visibility of ovarian morphology; hence, cleaning of the image is a requirement without hampering the necessary anatomical structures in the image (Mienye et al., 2025). Traditionally, noise-filtering and morphological methods fail to preserve the structural details important for accurate diagnosis, whereas deep learning-based denoising models, such as autoencoders and attention-based architectures, are better at reconstructing clearer images without affecting clinically relevant structures like follicles, cysts, and tissue boundaries. In addition, by learning discriminative features that distinguish healthy from pathological tissues, deep learning enables automated image analysis. For example, YOLO is an object detection algorithm suitable for locating anatomical structures and abnormalities in real-time systems, while classification models such as ResNet, DenseNet, and SE-enhanced networks can identify disease conditions with high accuracy. The automated models assist clinicians in their work and at the same time reduce the discrepancy between the interpretation of a clinician thereby improving the medical results and increasing their consistency. Explainable AI (XAI) is a new set of techniques in medical imaging, which leverages deep learning and represents an important advancement in the field (Pan et al., 2025). The Grad-CAM technique creates a clear picture by showing what parts of the image have affected the output of the model. The interpretability is to produce trusted output on the part of which the clinicians will trust it and administer the appropriate medication to the patients. The technology, such as deep learning, has demonstrated to be a spectacular and game-changing medical imaging tool by creating highly accurate automated diagnostic systems that are accessible on a large-scale basis. Deep learning facilitates the early detection of disease and clinical decision-making by merging data-driven feature extraction techniques, trusted pattern detection tools, and interpretable tools. Deep learning is needed to integrate data-driven feature learning, effective pattern recognition and interpretability to enable the early detection of diseases, clinical decision support, and design of personalized healthcare. Combining noise removal and follicle detection and ovarian classification and model interpretability through deep learning enables it to be a critical component of the healthcare system in the present day (Y. Zhang et al., 2021).

3.1.2 Role of Deep Learning in Ultrasound-Based Diagnosis

Ultrasound imaging is the diagnostic imaging technique that is most common. This technology can be used clinically due to the reasons that it is cheap, has real time image, and is portable in nature and can be used safely. The advantages of ultrasonic imaging are not without speckle noise, shadows, low contrast, and operator-related results. The limitation lowers the medical imaging diagnostic accuracy due to the hazy images of anatomy features. Deep learning(DL) can be helpful to address these challenges and improve the quality of the ultrasound imaging diagnostic (Zhou et al., 2025). Raw ultrasound images enjoy the advantages of deep learning models which rely on Convolutional Neural Networks (CNNs) and their more sophisticated forms to identify important characteristics. Deep learning models are independent of the human factor and can identify key features within the images. The models are superior in managing the natural intricacies of the ultrasound data. Deep learning in ultrasound diagnosis has the primary role of image enhancement and denoising. The autoencoders combined with attention-based networks allow to reduce the speckle noise successfully and retain significant clinical structures. It becomes possible to remove noise of images and hence detect small cysts, micro-lesions, and follicular patterns. Object detection models like YOLO, Faster R-CNN, and their descendants could be effectively used in a real-time system to detect regionally localized problems, including tumors, follicles, nodules, or lesions, in deep learning. It assists clinicians to have a consistent and objective localization and decrease the use of manual interpretation. The diagnosis of pathological conditions is another important Deep Learning input to ultrasound-based diagnosis. Deep learning architectures like ResNet, DenseNet, and SE-ResNet can be used to distinguish between normal and abnormal tissue patterns with high capabilities due to their capability to represent features in high-dimensional space (Mienye et al., 2025). Based on Deep Learning (DL)-based classifiers have also provided better performance over traditional machine-learning models as they can provide faster and more dependable results over diseases like Polycystic Ovary Syndrome (PCOS), thyroid nodules, breast cancer, and liver abnormalities. Besides these methods, another Explainable AI (XAI) method, like Grad-CAM, is another way of improving clinical application of deep learning systems. The concept of interpretability is extremely significant in the medical field where it is crucial to justify diagnostic recommendations in a clinical manner. Deep learning also facilitates repetition and uniformity in the diagnosis of ultrasound because, in case of heatmaps, the radiologist can understand which regions are contributing to the prediction (R. Yang et al., 2025). Since acquisition of ultrasound is highly subjective, clinicians might interpret ultrasound differently. DL models minimize this variability by offering standardized, automated assessment, enhancing diagnostic reliability between different practitioners and between different institutions. Deep learning has enhanced the ultrasound-based diagnostics to increase the image quality, identify anatomical structures, automatically classify diseases, and simplify the interpretation of the results. Modern medical imaging relies on it to extract meaningful information from noisy, variable ultrasound data. Ultrasound diagnostics, including applications such as PCOS detection, will benefit from advances in deep learning in the coming years, enabling earlier, more accurate, and less error-prone diagnosis (Dan et al., 2024).

3.1.3 Importance of Theoretical Foundations

Theoretical underpinnings are the base for creating, implementing, and interpreting deep learning-based models. Also, in complex diagnostic tasks such as ultrasound-based disease detection, a solid conceptual understanding is required to enable advanced algorithms to be implemented correctly, evaluated, interpreted, and validated in a clinical setting. The theoretical knowledge reflects the principles behind deep learning techniques. Concepts that make the backbone of the neural networks are convolution operations, activation functions, backpropagation, feature hierarchies, attention mechanisms, and residual learning, etc. hence without having knowledge of these fundamental concepts, it is very difficult to understand how models extract features, learn spatial patterns, or mitigate issues such as vanishing gradients (Mienye et al., 2025). A model design that is structured logically, rather than developed through trial-and-error experimentation, can only be ensured with a strong theoretical foundation. When selecting appropriate techniques, a theoretical concept plays an important role, based on the characteristics of the problem to be solved. The impurities that exist in ultrasound pictures are noise, low contrast, and variability, which need to be removed, and the models need to be chosen carefully. For example, if one knows about autoencoders, they can be used in the denoising process, while knowledge of multi-scale feature fusion explains why models like YOLOv8 are shown to be efficient at detecting variable-sized structures such as ovarian follicles (Shobayo & Saatchi, 2025). Theoretical knowledge also assists in justifying the reasons as to why a particular architecture is to be used on a particular issue. Theoretical foundations also guide the processes of model optimization and performance improvement. The understanding of the functioning of loss functions, optimization algorithms, and regularization techniques can help researchers tailor their models. Theoretical knowledge about these concepts can be used to perform the appropriate management of training issues like overfitting, class imbalance, and convergence instabilities that frequently occur with medical imaging data sets. Besides that, in the medical profession, deployment becomes ethical and responsible because of a theoretical foundation. Awareness of prejudices, generalizations, and dependence on data will create a way to avoid misinterpretation, which will make sure that models remain resilient between patients and imaging equipment. The variability in the way acquisition is performed influences the model in ultrasound imaging. Consequently, the theoretical underpinnings give substantial scientific intercourse and formulated justification of methods, which assist researchers to justify their methodological decisions in critique of how they did it in studies they have conducted in the past and add to scholarly discourse. Consequently, the study can be replicated and comprehended by other scientists in future. Therefore, theoretical underpinnings are important because they offer conceptual clarity, methodological choices, maximization of models, increased interpretability, ethical implementation, and academic integrity, and a theoretical basis of any deep learning based medical imaging study, to be able to convert its clinical utility and scientifically sound results.

3.2 FUNDAMENTALS OF DEEP LEARNING

Deep learning is employed to model complex and high dimensional data, which is a branch of machine learning that places more emphasis on artificial neural networks in multiple layers. Due to the automatic hierarchical-representation learning, it is regarded as one of the most successful methods in the contemporary artificial intelligence, particularly in processing pictures, sounds, and language. Deep learning models have transformed the foundations of diagnostic workflows by making possible a very high accuracy of prescription of complex visual patterns which were difficult to be analyzed by traditional algorithms when studying medical images.

The concept of deep learning is grounded on the functionality of the human brain and the connection between the neurons to one another in order to analyze and transmit information. The higher the layer, the more abstract manners the representation of things acquires. These layers tend to isolate low-level features like edges, textures, and forms. Lower layers, however, store higher level concepts like anatomical structures, pathogenic patterns or disease specific features. A deep learning network is trained by adjusting its parameters with the help of large datasets by the process of backpropagation. Through training the model repeatedly updates the weights and biases to minimize the difference between predictions and the true labels. Deep learning can be applied to ultrasonic imaging effectively due to the ability to enhance the internal representations automatically without features engineering. This is significant since noise, unpredictability, and ambiguity may result in difficulty in extracting features. Convolutional Neural Networks (CNNs) are a branch of deep learning, created to be applied primarily to spatial data, namely images. The CNN is an outstanding performer in classification, segmentation as well as object recognition due to the fact that it identifies the local image patterns as well as the spatial relationships thus performing outstandingly in the three activities. This is combined with the use of pooling layers so as to minimize the amount of computation as well as increase translational invariance. The activation functions in the deep learning models are necessary to add nonlinear relationships that allow the activation functions to learn complex patterns. ReLU, Sigmoid, and Tanh are considered as the three most frequently used functions of activation in the deep learning field. The neural networks are flexible and robust enough to learn complex patterns using nonlinear activation functions that are very useful in supporting a large variety of functions. The deep learning approach to medical imaging data set sets needs several regularization schemes to avoid overfitting on small datasets. The dropout, batch normalization, and data augmentation together allows the models to have better generalization through stability and robustness.

Deep learning models are now capable of extracting meaningful features of ultrasound images due to the invention of Residual Networks (ResNet), autoencoders, attention mechanisms and transformers. These are the three main problems that are dealt with by the three architectural designs, namely: vanishing gradients, insufficient training data, and absence of interpretability. Loss functions and optimization algorithms are also required to make deep learning models work. Medical imaging Deep learning models have the capability to perform simple classification tasks, more intricate tasks, including denoising, localization of anatomical structure and scaffolding images using Grad-CAM. The ultrasound systems with deep learning technology will be improved in diagnostic characteristics. The major aspect of the creation of advanced models of ultrasound image interpretation is the concept of deep learning because it provides both theoretical frameworks and computational procedures. Deep learning plays a key role in the current research in medical imaging since researchers can create the architecture to identify noise and control more delicate pathological ways and inter-rater variability in medical images. The invention of Residual Networks (ResNet), autoencoders, attention, and transformers has enabled deep learning models to extract significant information in ultrasound images. These architectural designs are aimed at addressing three issues: vanishing gradients, scarce training data and lack of interpretability. Deep learning models need optimization algorithms and loss functions in order to be functional. Simple tasks such as image classification and complex tasks such as noise reduction, location of body structures, and formation of new images using Grad-CAM are among the functions that medical imaging deep learning models will be able to perform with technology of deep learning. Deep learning also allows creating complex ultrasound image interpretation models by offering theoretical bases and computation. Deep learning is vital to the modern medical imaging research because researchers are able to create architectures that identify noise and can manipulate subtle pathological characteristics and variability in medical images.

3.2.1 Artificial Neural Networks (ANNs)

The foundation of deep learning is the artificial neural networks or ANNs. The human brain is a cluster of units known as neurons and they work together to find patterns on data available. Besides simple computation, in large, layered networks, the neurons can estimate complex functions, and are therefore very applicable in tasks such as classification, regression, pattern recognition, and analysis of medical images.

The ANN usually has three layers, i.e., input, hidden, and output. Raw data are fed into the input layer e.g. pixel intensities on an ultrasound image. Computations are done in the hidden layers with intermediate computations being made and the abstract features being extracted whilst the output layer creates the final prediction which could be a probability score which indicates the presence or absence of a condition like PCOS. The inputs are also multiplied by weights associated with them and then a bias term is added to the result which is then subjected to an activation function in artificial neurons. The fundamental calculation that is carried out by a neuron is given as:

$$y = f\left(\sum_{i=1}^{n} \omega_i \chi_i + b\right) \tag{1}$$

where,

- x_i are input values,
- w_i are weights,
- b is the bias,
- f is the activation function,
- y i s the neuron's output

3.2.1.1 Activation Functions

The use of activation functions makes networks become nonlinear, enabling them to acquire complex, nonlinear relationships. The following activation functions are as follows:

- **Sigmoid:**

$$\sigma(x) = \frac{1}{1 + e^{-x}} \tag{2}$$

- **Tanh (Hyperbolic Tangent):**

$$\tanh(x) = \frac{e^x - e^{-x}}{e^x + e^{-x}} \tag{3}$$

- **ReLU (Rectified Linear Unit):**

$$f(x) = \max(0, x) \quad (4)$$

Being widely used, ReLU reduces vanishing gradients and makes deep networks simple.

3.2.1.2 Learning Process in ANNs

Artificial neural networks (ANNs) are trained to change their weights and biases to minimize the difference between actual and desired outputs. This training involves loss functions (such as mean squared error and cross-entropy loss), optimization algorithms (such as gradient descent and Adam) and backpropagation, which calculates how to change the weights and Backpropagation uses the chain rule to propagate error signals backward through the network. This approach allows learning efficiently even in case the model contains many parameters. Artificial neural networks have various types of structures; the following are some of them:

(i) **Feedforward Neural Networks (FNNs):** Feedforward signals run only in one direction; this type is very popular as a simple classifier.

(ii) **Recurrent Neural Networks (RNNs):** It is structured to adapt to sequential data, which is appropriate in time-series analysis.

(iii) **Radial Basis Function Networks (RBFNs):** The radial functions are used as an activation; they are useful in interpolation.

Among these three categories of medical imaging, the feed-forward networks are the most constructive as they can be used to form more advanced models, including convolutional neural networks (CNNs), autoencoders, and residual networks (ResNets).

3.2.1.3 Relevance of ANNs in Medical Imaging

The initial move towards the automation of the analysis of medical image was artificial neural networks (ANNs). Even though nowadays the convolutional designs are more often used in applications, artificial neural networks (ANNs) remain topical because of their theoretical contribution to:

a) Networks learning data.
b) The effects of parameters on prediction.
c) How are the errors reduced in the process of training?

Such methods are still relevant in the high-level ultrasonic analysis, such as deep autoencoders, attention models, object detectors.

3.2.2 Deep Neural Networks (DNNs)

Deep Neural Networks (DNNs) are a more complicated form of the Artificial Neural Networks(ANNs) that is defined by a number of hidden layers between the input and the resulting output. As a rule, standard artificial neural networks (ANNs) would include one or two hidden layers, and deep neural networks (DNNs) have a far deeper structure. This gives rise to deep neural networks capable of learning complicated, abstract, and nonlinear patterns of the data. The complexity of Deep Neural Networks (DNNs) enables them to capture multidimensional relationships and they can therefore be extremely useful in applications like recognizing images, analyzing audio, natural language processing, and imaging which are, in turn, very helpful in the medical field. A simple pattern, edges, and simple gradient are simple attributes which the model is being taught to identify at the first stages of deep neural networks (DNNs). Then more intricate structures are discovered on the middle levels, including shapes or textures. Finally, the deep-layers are the ones that detect high-level semantic patterns e.g., organs, lesions and other abnormalities. According to the fundamental concepts of the artificial neural networks (ANNs) Deep Neural Networks (DNNs) are defined by their hierarchical nature of extracting information.

3.2.2.1 Architecture of DNNs

The elements of the Deep neural networks are as follows:

(i) **Input Layer**
(ii) **Multiple Hidden Layers**
(iii)**Output Layer**

The input layer receives raw data, for example, ultrasound pixel values. Multiple hidden layers perform sequential nonlinear transformations through weighted connections, activations, and normalization, and the output layer produces the final predictions, such as the probability of the disease being present. The transformation performed in each hidden layer can be mathematically expressed as:

$$h^{(l)} = f\left(W^{(l)}h^{(l-1)} + b^{(l)}\right) \tag{5}$$

where,

- $\boldsymbol{h}^{(l)}$ is the output of the l-th layer,
- $\boldsymbol{W}^{(l)}$& $\boldsymbol{b}^{(l)}$= weight matrix and bias vector
- $\boldsymbol{f}(\cdot)$= activation function

Hence, Deep neural networks (DNNs) can estimate very complex functions because of their many layers, which makes them universal function approximators.

Deep Neural Networks(DNNs) are trained using following components which are as follows:

(i) **Loss Functions** like cross-entropy, MSE, etc.
(ii) **Optimization Algorithms** like SGD, Adam, etc.

(iii)**Backpropagation Algorithm**, which updates model parameters by computing gradients layer-by-layer.

On the other hand, deeper networks face several obstacles, such as **vanishing or exploding gradients, overfitting on small datasets, and High computational demand.** ResNets, Batch normalization, dropout regularization, and Weight initialization techniques are examples of advances that resulted from this. The progress of the far more powerful models is that they are able to generalize better and to converge more easily, especially in medical imaging tasks where the quantity of data at hand may be limited. DNNs have a number of benefits that can be specifically applied to medical imaging and include:

1. Hierarchical Feature Learning: This method is necessary in medical imaging in order to avoid all the differences which was not evident in the conventional methods. In this case, DNNs are very important, which automatically identify Texture, Shape, Lesion boundaries, and abnormal tissue patterns.

2. Stability to Noise: Ultrasound images have anomalies such as speckle noise and artifacts.DNNs are trained to have representations that are invariant to noise, and that maintain their important structure.

3. High Accuracy in Classification and Detection: The systems that are DNN-based outperform traditional machine learning models in identifying PCOS patterns, Tumors, Nodules, and Organ abnormalities.

4. Adaptability to Multiple Tasks: DNNs can be adapted for Denoising, Segmentation, Classification, Localization, and Interpretability (with XAI methods).

3.2.2.2 Relevance of DNNs to Ultrasound-Based PCOS Diagnosis

In the context of ultrasound imaging for PCOS, **DNN-based autoencoders** help remove speckle noise; deep convolutional layers identify follicles, cysts, and ovarian structures; deep classifiers distinguish PCOS ovaries from normal ones using subtle features; **and Attention-based deep networks** further enhance performance by focusing on diagnostic regions. Hence, this makes DNNs an essential theoretical foundation for your research work.

3.2.2.3 Convolutional Neural Networks (CNNs)

Convolutional Neural Networks (CNNs) are a specialized type of deep neural network designed primarily to process grid-like data, such as images. Convolutional Neural Networks (CNNs) have become the primary architecture in computer vision because they can automatically learn spatial hierarchies of features, from basic edges to complex patterns, without requiring manually engineered feature extraction methods. Therefore, the ability of CNNs to recognise small differences in structures and textures makes them especially useful in medical imaging, where these features are vital for accurate diagnosis. Unlike typical fully connected networks, CNNs employ convolutional operations. This approach greatly reduces the number of parameters to train while preserving the spatial connections within the image. This approach not only increases computational efficiency but also boosts the reliability of convolutional neural networks (CNNs) for medical applications, such as detecting polycystic ovary syndrome (PCOS) using ultrasonography.

3.2.2.4 Convolution Operation

Convolution, the main operation of a Convolutional Neural Network (CNN), involves a small, trainable matrix called a kernel or filter. This kernel is applied to the input images to create feature maps. This helps the network to identify the local patterns.

Mathematically, the convolution operation can be defined as:

$$F(i,j) = \sum_{m} \sum_{n} I(i+m, j+n) \cdot K(m,n) \tag{6}$$

where ,

- ***I*** is the input image
- ***K*** is the convolutional kernel
- ***F*** is the resulting feature map.

Convolutions capture important visual features like edges, corners, textures and patterns related to follicles, cysts, or lesions.

3.2.2.5 Activation Functions

After convolution, activation functions introduce non-linearity, enabling CNNs to model complex medical patterns.

Common activation functions include:

(i) **ReLU (Rectified Linear Unit)**

$$f(x) = \max(0, x) \tag{7}$$

(ii) **Leaky ReLU**: It addresses the dead neuron problem.
(iii)**Sigmoid** and **Tanh**: It is mainly used in output layers or specialized cases.

3.2.2.6 Pooling Layers

The process of pooling decreases the spatial dimensions of feature maps keeping the most significant information. The kinds of pooling are as follows:

i. Max Pooling (most widespread): This picks the best value in the area; works with images that have a lot of texture such as ultrasound.
ii. Average Pooling: It uses the mean; applied in the global pooling to classify it.

Some of the advantages of pooling are lower computation, translation invariance, avoiding overfitting and extraction of the dominant.

3.2.2.7 Feature Maps and Hierarchical Representation

Convolutional neural networks (CNNs) are trained in hierarchical features, and they are as follows:

i. Early layers: It identifies lines, corners, and edges.
ii. Middle layers: It identifies textures, shapes and anatomical outlines.
iii. Deep layers: It identifies abstract features including ovarian morphology or cluster of cysts.

Such hierarchy is important to medical imaging where slight abnormalities need to be differentiated with normal tissue textures.

3.2.2.8 Padding and Stride

Padding maintains a spatial resolution by inserting zeros around the input and Stride is the distance that the kernel runs over the image. These are parameters that regulate the size of the feature map of output and detail of capture.

3.2.2.9 Fully Connected Layers

In CNNs towards the end, the extracted features are combined into fully connected (FC) layers to classify them:

$$y = softmax(Wx + b) \quad (8)$$

In medical imaging, FC layers transform extracted features to probabilities of being diseased.

3.2.3.0 CNN Advantages in Medical Imaging

The CNNs are popular because of a number of advantages:

i. **Automatic Feature Extraction:** Abandons the manual feature engineering that is essential in ultrasound, where patterns are delicate.
ii. **Spatial Awareness:** Its conserves the local anatomical structures.
iii. **Resistance to Noise:** It is paramount that ultrasound images with speckle noise.
iv. **Scalability:** It is able to do complex processes such as denoising, segmentation, classification and object detection.
v. **High-accuracy:** CNNs are always identified as more accurate than the conventional ML methods in detecting diseases.

3.2.3.1 Relevance of CNNs in Ultrasound-Based PCOS Diagnosis

CNNs would be the most appropriate method of PCOS detection in ultrasound imaging as they can detect follicle borders, cyst patterns, ovarian morphology, automated follicle counting, and distinguish between normal and polycystic patterns. ResNets based on CNNs are also used in the ResNet, SE-ResNet, Autoencoders, YOLO detection backbone, Feature extraction modules, and Grad-CAM interpretations. Thus, all the deep learning methods applied in PCOS research rely on CNNs as their base. The process of pooling makes feature maps smaller hence it conserves most important information. Pooling reduces the size of feature maps, which helps preserve the most critical information.

3.2.3 Optimization Algorithms (SGD, Adam)

Deep learning models rely on optimization algorithms which modify the parameters of the network in the course of training. These algorithms operate by the repeated adaptation of weights and biases to optimize the loss function, and thus decrease the error in prediction. Good convergence, faster learning and improved generalization depends on good optimization. All these are significant in medical imaging whereby the quality and quantity of data may vary. Optimization in deep learning Minimization of a problem:

In deep learning, optimization involves addressing a minimization problem :

$$\min_{\theta} L(\theta) \quad (9)$$

where,

- $\boldsymbol{\theta}$ represents model parameters (weights and biases)
- $\boldsymbol{L(\theta)}$ is the loss function measuring prediction error.

Stochastic Gradient Descent (SGD) and Adam are the two most popular optimization algorithms in the field of deep learning, both of which are necessary in the process of training the models to be applied in medical ultrasonography analysis.

3.2.4 Stochastic Gradient Descent (SGD)

Stochastic Gradient Descent (SGD) is a data representation technique that produces a series of random samples based on the current data. One of the most elementary, as well as widely used optimization methods, is Stochastic Gradient Descent. This technique updates the model parameters using small data sets instead of full sets. This results in better computational effectiveness.

The SGD mathematical expression is as follows:

$$\theta_{t+1} = \theta_t - \eta \cdot \nabla_\theta L(\theta_t) \tag{10}$$

where ,

- $\boldsymbol{\eta}$= learning rate
- $\boldsymbol{\nabla_\theta L(\theta_t)}$= gradient of the loss function with respect to parameters
- $\boldsymbol{t}$= iteration index

Advantages of SGD

(i) It is computationally efficient.
(ii) It works well for large datasets.
(iii)The faster updates improve model responsiveness.

Limitations of SGD

(i) It is sensitive to the learning rate.
(ii) It can get trapped in local minima.
(iii)It has slow convergence for noisy gradients.
(iv)It may struggle with complex loss surfaces typical in medical imaging networks.

SGD with Momentum

Momentum is an improvement to Stochastic Gradient Descent (SGD) that speeds up the learning process by adding a velocity term:

$$v_{t+1} = \gamma v_t + \eta \cdot \nabla_\theta L(\theta_t) \tag{11}$$

$$\theta_{t+1} = \theta_t - v_{t+1} \tag{12}$$

where ,

$\boldsymbol{\gamma}$ = momentum coefficient (typically 0.9)

Momentum helps the algorithm to smoothly traverse ravines, to avoid oscillations, and speed up convergence.

3.2.5 Adam (Adaptive Moment Estimation)

Adam has become a go-to optimizer in deep learning, particularly in medical imaging. This method combines the strengths of Momentum and RMSProp by using an adaptive learning rate for each parameter. Adam calculates two moment estimates, which are as follows:

(i) **First Moment (Mean of Gradients):**

$$m_t = \beta_1 m_{t-1} + (1 - \beta_1)\nabla_\theta L(\theta_t) \tag{13}$$

(ii) **Second Moment (Uncentered Variance of Gradients):**

$$v_t = \beta_2 v_{t-1} + (1 - \beta_2)\left(\nabla_\theta L(\theta_t)\right)^2 \tag{14}$$

To correct initialization bias, Adam uses bias-corrected estimates:

$$\hat{m}_t = \frac{m_t}{1 - \beta_1^t}, \hat{v}_t = \frac{v_t}{1 - \beta_2^t} \tag{15}$$

Finally, the parameter update rule is:

$$\theta_{t+1} = \theta_t - \eta \cdot \frac{\hat{m}_t}{\sqrt{\hat{v}_t} + \epsilon} \tag{16}$$

where,

- $\boldsymbol{\beta_1} = \mathbf{0.9}$, $\boldsymbol{\beta_2} = 0.999$(default values)
- $\boldsymbol{\epsilon \approx 10^{-8}}$ for numerical stability

3.2.6 Advantages of Adam

Adam possesses various attributes that render it well-suited for deep learning applications in medical imaging, which are as follows :

(i) **Adaptive learning rates:** Here, each parameter adjusts individually.
(ii) **Fast convergence:** It works well for noisy or sparse gradients.
(iii)**Low memory requirement**: Compared to second-order methods, it takes low memory space.
(iv)**Stable training**: Even on small and noisy medical datasets, it trains well.
(v) **Excellent performance:** In models having attention blocks, autoencoders, and CNNs, it gives excellent performance.

These advantages explain why Adam is commonly used to train denoising networks, detection models such as YOLO, and classification networks such as SE-ResNet for ultrasound-based diagnostics. Adam usually performs better than other methods when applied to complex deep learning models in medical imaging. However, Stochastic gradient descent (SGD) with momentum could generalize better for some large-scale applications.

3.2.7 Relevance to Ultrasound-Based PCOS Detection

Optimization algorithms directly influence the training stability, noise robustness, detection accuracy, classification performance, and convergence speed. Both **SGD** and **Adam** ensure effective learning for models such as Autoencoders (denoising), CNN-based classifiers, ResNet/SE-ResNet, YOLOv8 detection models, and Attention-enhanced architectures. Therefore, a strong grasp of optimization methods is important for developing and training deep learning systems for ultrasound image processing.

3.2.8 Loss Functions Overview

The deep learning models cannot be complete without loss functions. They can be used as mathematical methods to determine the error between the predicted output of a network and the correct answer provided. The key aim of the optimization algorithm during the training process is to reduce the loss by changing the parameters of the model. The selection of a loss function is important because it has a direct influence on the learning behavior of the model, its convergence speed, stability, and its overall performance. This is particularly crucial in medical imaging where accuracy and reliability are crucial. Loss functions control the network learning by showing the goodness of prediction. This input can be propagated backward through the network using Backpropagation to assist the optimizer in the process of modifying weights and biases. The classification, regression, object detection, and image denoising tasks involve different loss functions given the differences in their output structures and the problem complexity. When performing ultrasonography to diagnose PCOS, a number of loss functions are usually used depending on the type of deep learning approach that is being used, e.g. denoising, classification or detection. The key functions of losses that are pertinent to the field of medicine imaging are as follows:

3.2.8.1 Mean Squared Error (MSE) Loss

Mean Squared Error is one of the most fundamental regression loss functions, and it's commonly used in image restoration and denoising tasks. The mathematical expression for finding the MSE loss is shown below:

$$L_{MSE} = \frac{1}{n}\sum_{i=1}^{n} (y_i - \hat{y}_i)^2 \tag{17}$$

where ,

- $\boldsymbol{y_i}$= ground truth pixel
- $\boldsymbol{\hat{y}_i}$= reconstructed pixel

MSE is used in medical imaging because it penalizes large errors, encouraging smoother reconstructions, suitable for denoising autoencoders, and is simple and differentiable. However, MSE may cause blurring since it averages errors across all pixels.

3.2.8.2 Mean Absolute Error (MAE) Loss

MAE calculates the average absolute difference between predictions and true values. It is mathematically expressed as follows:

$$\boldsymbol{L_{MAE}} = \frac{\mathbf{1}}{\boldsymbol{n}}\sum_{\boldsymbol{i=1}}^{\boldsymbol{n}} \mid \boldsymbol{y_i} - \boldsymbol{\hat{y}_i} \mid \tag{18}$$

The main advantage of using MAE is that it is more robust to outliers than MSE and Preserves edges better in medical images. MAE is useful when the model must avoid over-smoothing.

3.2.8.3 Binary Cross-Entropy (BCE) Loss

Binary Cross Entropy (BCE) is used for binary classification tasks, such as identifying normal vs. PCOS ovaries. Mathematically, it is expressed as :

$$L_{BCE} = -[y\log(\hat{y}) + (1-y)\log(1-\hat{y})] \tag{19}$$

where ,

- y= true label (0 or 1)
- $\hat{y}$= predicted probability

There are several benefits that exist, like it is Ideal for sigmoid outputs, encouraging probability calibration, and being effective for clinical classification tasks.

3.2.8.4 Categorical Cross-Entropy Loss

It is used when the classification involves multiple classes. The mathematical expression for the same is :

$$L_{CCE} = -\sum_{c=1}^{C} y_c \log(\hat{y}_c) \tag{20}$$

where ,

- C= number of classes,
- y_c= one-hot encoded true label

- $\hat{y}_c$= predicted probability for class c

3.2.8.5 Dice Loss

Dice Loss is specifically designed for segmentation tasks in medical imaging. Mathematically, it is expressed as :

$$L_{Dice} = 1 - \frac{2 \mid X \cap Y \mid}{\mid X \mid + \mid Y \mid} \tag{21}$$

where ,

- X= predicted region
- Y= actual region

Dice Loss is important because it is useful for imbalanced datasets, focuses on region overlap, and encourages accurate boundary detection.

3.2.8.6 IoU (Intersection-over-Union) Loss

IoU Loss is used in object detection models like YOLO to ensure accurate bounding box localization. It is mathematically expressed as follows:

$$L_{IoU} = 1 - IoU \tag{22}$$

$$IoU = \frac{\mid A \cap B \mid}{\mid A \cup B \mid} \tag{23}$$

3.2.8.7 Focal Loss

Focal Loss addresses class imbalance by reducing the loss contribution of well-classified examples. It is mathematically expressed as follows:

$$L_{Focal} = -\alpha(1 - \hat{y})^{\gamma} log\ (\hat{y}) \quad (24)$$

where ,

- γ Controls focus on difficult cases
- α balances class distribution

3.2.8.8 Combined or Composite Loss Functions

Many deep learning models used in medical imaging employ composite loss functions to maximise multiple goals simultaneously.

For example (for a denoising autoencoder), the mathematical expression is :

$$L = L_{MSE} + \lambda L_{regularization} \quad (25)$$

For Example (for detection models), the mathematical expression is :

$$L = L_{classification} + L_{localization} + L_{confidence} \quad (26)$$

Composite losses ensure balanced learning between tasks such as Denoising quality, Object localization, and feature discrimination.

3.2.8.9 Relevance of Loss Functions in Ultrasound-Based PCOS Diagnosis

In PCOS diagnosis using ultrasound images, MAE has been used for autoencoder-based speckle noise reduction, Cross-Entropy has been used for classification of PCOS vs. normal ovaries, IoU / GIoU / Focal Loss has been used in follicle detection (YOLO models), and Regularization losses have been used for preventing overfitting on limited medical datasets. Selecting the appropriate loss function ensures better convergence, more accurate detection, Robust classification, enhanced interpretability, and clinically reliable performance. Hence, loss functions are a critical theoretical component of deep learning based medical imaging systems.

3.3 AUTOENCODERS

Autoencoders are a form of unsupervised deep learning model that is employed in the generation of small, informative representations of data. This is done through the reconstruction of the input at the output layer once it is coded into a smaller hidden representation. Autoencoders are common in medical imaging in applications like denoising, feature extraction, anomaly detection, dimensionality reduction. These approaches are very effective in analysing complex and noisy ultrasound images because they are able to identify the patterns of data.

3.3.1 Concept and Architecture

The main aim of an autoencoder is to create an efficient persona of input data with minimum noise and redundancy, just as much as important information is retained. The overall design with encoder and decoder modules is connected to each other via the latent space representation otherwise referred to as a bottleneck. Training the model to push the network to capture the key characteristics in the latent space the model works to reduce the reconstruction error between the original input and the reconstruction.

3.3.2 Encoder

The encoder represents the input data in a low-dimensional form. It minimizes the use of space and removes successively more abstract features by applying a large number of transformations typically using convolutional or fully connected layers.

If $\boldsymbol{x}$ represents the input image, the encoder performs:

$$z = f_{encoder}(x) \tag{27}$$

where,

- $\boldsymbol{z}$= latent vector
- $\boldsymbol{f_{encoder}}$= transformation function which is composed of learnable weights and activation functions. Encoders in medical imaging detect patterns that include boundaries, textures, follicles shapes and morphology of organs.

3.3.3 Latent Space Representation

Latent space or the bottleneck layer is the compressed vector representing the most important information extracted out of the input. It is a low-dimensional embedding that expresses the structure and the variability of the data. The features of a good latent representation are low redundancy, high information density, usefulness in reconstructing key features and anti-noise and distortion. In the case of ultrasound, the latent space is able to capture important data about anatomy and exclude redundant textual distractions.

3.3.4 Decoder

The decoder is identical to the encoder but it does the reverse task of blowing the latent vector back to the original data dimensions.

It performs:

$$\hat{x} = f_{decoder}(z) \tag{28}$$

where,

$\hat{x}$= reconstructed image

The decoder guarantees recovery of critical structures, maintenance of spatial patterns and accuracy of reconstruction. The decoder is also highly important in the denoising applications as it generates a cleaner image and less speckle noise without loss of other diagnostic information.

3.3.5 Variants of Autoencoders

A number of autoencoders variants have been created to deal with particular learning tasks or limitations. There are two types that are important in medical imaging and they are as follows:

3.3.6 Denoising Autoencoders (DAE)

Denoising Autoencoders are made to eliminate noise in corrupted data. The training is performed by corrupting the input image artificially:

$$x_{noisy} = x + noise \tag{29}$$

The objective of the model is:

$$\hat{x} = f(x_{noisy}) \tag{30}$$

These models are trained on how to recover clean ultrasound images based on noisy images. This is particularly crucial in ultrasound imaging; speckle noise dramatically diminishes diagnostic imaging. Speckle noise removal, retention of follicular structures, and increased visibility of cysts are the advantages of DAE usage.

3.3.7 Sparse Autoencoders

Sparse Autoencoders are based on sparsity in the latent space. It is a process that only a few neurons are active and assist in the process of extracting specific features. The sparsity promotes model to learn different structural properties, clean representations and semantics at higher levels. The reason why these autoencoders are effective in preventing overfitting is because these autoencoders are applied to small datasets, as is often the case in medical ultrasound studies. It is assumed that the autoencoder is composed of an encoder function fand a decoder function **g.**

(i) **Encoding Step:**

$$z = f(x) = \sigma(W_e x + b_e) \tag{31}$$

(ii) **Decoding Step:**

$$\hat{x} = g(z) = \sigma(W_d z + b_d) \tag{32}$$

The reconstruction loss function, typically Mean Squared Error (MSE), is:

$$L(x, \hat{x}) = \| x - \hat{x} \|^2 \tag{33}$$

The other regularizers are Sparsity constraints, weight penalties, and attention regularization. These regularization techniques ensure that the model learns compact, meaningful embeddings.

3.3.8 Applications in Image Denoising

Autoencoders are widely used in medical imaging for denoising tasks, as they can distinguish meaningful structures from noise. In Ultrasound Imaging, Autoencoders can be used for noise removal, image clarity enhancement, preservation of organ boundaries, and improved feature variability for diagnostic models. Autoencoders Improve Denoising :

(i) Encoder learns abstract, noise-free representations
(ii) Decoder reconstructs clean images
(iii)The network learns to ignore random noise patterns
(iv)Latent space filters out irrelevant textures

Benefits of PCOS Diagnosis:

(i) Enhancing visibility of ovarian follicles
(ii) Avoids loss of diagnostic information
(iii)Improves downstream tasks such as follicle detection and classification

3.4 ATTENTION MECHANISMS

Attention mechanisms help deep learning models focus on the most important features in images or sequences. In medical imaging, particularly when using ultrasound-based PCOS detection, attention improves interpretability and improves model accuracy by guiding the network toward clinically relevant regions, such as follicles or ovarian boundaries.

3.4.1 Need for Attention in Deep Models

Deep CNNs are designed to extract characteristics in a hierarchical way. However, they also have several drawbacks, which are loss of spatial information due to pooling layers, difficulty identifying small or irregular structures (e.g., follicles in PCOS), equal weighting of all features, even when some regions are irrelevant, and **poor interpretability**. Attention mechanisms address these issues by highlighting important regions and suppressing noise, thereby improving feature representation, enhancing explainability, and supporting fine-grained medical image tasks such as segmentation and detection. **In PCOS imaging**, attention helps the model focus on follicle clusters, ovarian stroma, cyst size and shape, and texture variations.

3.4.2 Spatial Attention

Spatial attention is a cognitive process that helps to concentrate on the relevant parts of an ultrasound image. It operates on **spatial dimensions** ($H \times W$), generates a spatial attention map indicating **important image locations**, helps detect localized structures like **small follicles**, and is often used alongside channel attention (e.g., in CBAM). The advantages of applying the spatial attention are that it is better in localizing the abnormalities and can be used in segmentation, disease detection, and ROI localization.

3.4.3 Channel Attention

Channel attention is centered on the most important aspects that are important on various channels. It does not work in spatial dimensions but in channels, it learns which channel encodes the most important features and it assists in highlighting features of texture, intensity and structure patterns. One has to do global average pooling and max pooling, pass through fully connected layers (MLP), compute channel attention weights, and multiply the weights by the input feature channels.

The following are some of the advantages of channel attention is:

(i) It improves discriminative features.

(ii) It is perfect in identifying subtle differences in texture of ultrasound images.

3.4.4 Self-Attention Concept

Each feature is given a chance to interact with the entire features in an image by self-attention and therefore, it is able to learn about the long-term relations. The fundamental principle of Transformers is to calculate similarity of pairs of features and acquire the entire context, unlike CNNs that concentrate on local neighbourhoods. The concept of self-attention is significant since ultrasound images are usually full of noises and overlapping structures and it also records the relationship between distant regions, which is better in detecting. Self-attention has many real-time applications: vision transformers (ViT), Swin Transformers, and hybrid CNNs in conjunction with Attention Models.

The Mathematical Representation of Attention is as follows:

Given queries **(Q)**, keys **(K)**, and values **(V)**:

$$\mathrm{Attention}(Q, K, V) = \mathrm{softmax}\left(\frac{QK^{T}}{\sqrt{d_k}}\right)V \tag{34}$$

where ,

- **Q** is the query matrix
- **K** is the key matrix
- **V** is a value matrix
- $\boldsymbol{d_k}$ is a dimension of keys, and softmax ensures attention weights sum to 1.

In this case, the attention mechanism computes the similarity with $\boldsymbol{QK^T}$ at the first stage, scales it with a $\sqrt{\boldsymbol{d_k}}$, and normalizes the scores with the help of a softmax activation function, followed by multiplication of the resultant weights with V to produce attended features. Through this process, the model may learn what pixels or areas in the image are correlated with other pixels or areas and learn to give more importance to areas that are important clinically.

3.4.5 Applications in Medical Imaging

The attention mechanisms have broad medical imaging applications in that they allow one to target the most informative areas in an image. It can be implied in several areas which are important. Attention is used in the classification of diseases to determine distinguishing regions, which can be used to detect an activity (e.g. PCOS). In segmentation, incorporation of attention gates in architectures like U-Net is used to improve the segmentation of tumor boundaries, organs, and follicles on the ovarian ultrasound images. Attention assists in the identification of more regions of interest (ROIs) to be able to detect and locate lesions, cysts and anatomical structures more precisely. Attention maps or heatmaps assist doctors in the explainability (XAI) process, making them observe what components of the model influence its predictions. These create the trust and aid doctors in decision making. Lastly, attention mechanisms in multimodal fusion are capable of combining the data of multiple sources, e.g. ultrasound and clinical data, MRI and CT, or text and imaging, etc., and making sure that the most relevant modality will have a greater role in the final prediction.

3.5 SPECKLE NOISE IN ULTRASOUND IMAGING

The noise that is prevalent and is inherent to the ultrasound imaging is known as the speckle noise. These artifacts present themselves in the form of small, gritty sets, which minimize the quality of pictures and blur important anatomical details. Speckle noise is not simply a noise; it is in fact a way of telling how the structure is. Nevertheless, it reduces contrast and visibility as well, thus complicating the medical image perception and its automatic analysis.

3.5.1 Nature of Speckle Noise

The speckle noise is as a result of the coherent nature of the ultrasound waves. The incoming ultrasound waves entering several small scatterers in the biological tissues give a returning wave that either sum or cancel in biological tissues. The wave pattern of interference gives an appearance of grainy look that is referred to as speckle. Strength of the signal determines how much multiplicative noise it will generate as the effect of noise is directly proportional to signal intensity. The intensity of the speckle patterns is greater in the high-intensity light areas and lesser in the low-intensity light areas. The distinct characteristic of the ultrasonic images is their look as compared to other medical images made by the other imaging methods.

3.5.2 Sources and Effects

The presence of a large number of small tissue interfaces which act as scatterers results in the creation of speckle noise. The reflections of the waves on the scatterers cause the wave to appear in random forms thus creating random variations in intensities. Speckle formation is affected by various factors such as the frequency of ultrasound image, the properties of the transducer and changes in tissue properties. The speckle noise increases the quality of images by making the images less clear and contrasted as well as obscuring minor anatomical details. The speckle noise makes matters more challenging in obtaining the clinical diagnosis of PCOS since speckle noise covers important characteristics, such as follicles, boundaries of cysts, and ovarian tissue appearances. Due to this effect, it is hard to measure the ovarian volume and the size of the follicles.

In the case of automated systems, the speckle noise impairs feature extraction and decreases the accuracy of segmentation and increases the probability of misclassification.

3.5.3 Mathematical Expression of Speckle Noise

In ultrasound imaging, speckle noise is often modelled as multiplicative noise. The observed degraded image $I(x, y)$is frequently represented as:

$$I(x, y) = S(x, y) \cdot N(x, y) \tag{35}$$

where ,

- $\boldsymbol{S(x, y)}$is the true underlying signal
- $\boldsymbol{N(x, y)}$is the speckle noise component.

Speckle noise can in most instances assume the Rayleigh, Gamma or Negative Exponential distribution based on the imaging conditions. The modeling is useful in designing filters and deep learning-based methods of denoising ultrasound images to classify them.

3.5.4 Challenges for Deep Learning Systems

Speckle noise reduction in image is subject to a number of challenges. In most cases, deep learning systems are likely to be confused with the speckle patterns and real anatomical structures and thus misinterpret data. Besides this, the introduction of noise raises the intra-class variability within each and every class. In its turn, this serves as an obstacle to the distinction of healthy and diseased ovarian tissue by the model. The existence of similarities in the overwhelming likelihood of distinguishing between normal and disease-setting ovarian tissues complicates the matter and makes it more challenging to differentiate the two by models. Strong speckle patterns hide important structural features and it is hard to allow models to learn meaningful representations in the presence of strong speckle patterns. This can lead to the situation where activities like segmentation, classification, and detection become inaccurate.

3.6 IMAGE DENOISING TECHNIQUES

Image denoising is also important in enhancing the quality of the ultrasound images by eliminating the noises associated with specularity without eliminating imperative details. The advantages of successful denoising are enhanced visibility, increased accuracy of the diagnoses, and enhanced completion of the deep learning models of the next task like segmentation and classification. The conventional denoising methods are dependent on heavy mathematical operations and filtering to eliminate noise in ultrasound images. The purpose of these filtering methods is to trade-off between noise reduction and edge and texture preservation and to locate structures such as ovarian follicles. The different methods of filters are described briefly as below:

3.6.1 Mean Filter

One of the techniques that remove noise is the mean filter that replaces each pixel with the average of the neighbouring pixels. In spite of the fact that this method is simple and computationally fast in comparison with other methods of filtering, it tends to cause too much blurring that may eliminate useful structural information in ultrasound images.

3.6.1.1 Median Filter

The median filter works based on the principle of the replacement of each pixel with the Neighbor median. The filtering method is especially appropriate in eliminating impulsive noise and it is more effective in maintaining edges of an image as compared to the mean filter. Although it could still be able to obscure vital details in medical imaging.

3.6.1.2 Gaussian Filter

The Gaussian filter is a filter that is used in order to smooth out images using a Gaussian kernel. It is a process that minimises high frequency noise and preserves edges. Although it is effective, this technique may blur sharp lines and minute details like a small follicle. The center functionality of the Gaussian filter is the smoothing of a picture comparing to a Gaussian Kernel.

3.6.1.3 Bilateral Filter

The bilateral filter eliminates noise of the images with keeping edges intact by taking into consideration the spatial proximity as well as the intensity difference between pixels. The dual-weighting technique enables even areas to be smooth and significant boundaries to be left. This is among the milestone reasons that the bilateral filtering is a popular medical imaging filter.

3.6.1.4 Wavelet-Based Denoising

Wavelet based denoising operates by converting the image into the wavelet domain where it is possible to isolate noise and the signal. Through thresholding of wavelet coefficients, noise may be minimized effectively and allow significant structural information to be preserved. The method is very effective in ultrasonic imaging since speckle noise is better addressed compared to spatial filters.

3.6.1.5 Non-Local Means (NLM)

The pixels that share similar intensity patterns are summed up by the Non-Local Means (NLM) filter irrespective of the geographical position to minimize noise in an image. This method is more effective and effective at keeping complex structures and fine textures, as compared to local filters. However, it is computationally costly especially on images that are of high quality in ultrasound.

3.6.2 Deep Learning Based Denoising

Deep learning-based image denoising can adaptively learn image content and is suitable for denoising tasks in high-noise environments. Image denoising has long been a research hotspot in image processing, aiming to remove noise from imaging devices, external environments, and other interfering factors to restore noisy images to their original, clean, noise-free state. Mature algorithms and machine learning techniques have been developed for various application scenarios and specific computer vision tasks (Z. Li, 2023).

3.7 OBJECT DETECTION TECHNIQUES

Object detection is a core challenge for computer vision. The process of object detection in images involves identifying and localizing objects using rectangular bounding box annotations. Medical imaging depends on object detection to detect both normal body structures and pathological lesions and abnormalities. The automated detection of ovarian structures, follicles, and cysts through object detection helps doctors perform better clinical assessments in ultrasound-based PCOS diagnosis (Tennekoon et al., 2025).

3.7.1 Introduction to Object Detection

Object detection is a combination of two significant features that include image classification and object localization.

The classification is used to identify the object that is in the image and the localization is used to identify the location of that object in the image. Object detection models today do this in a single step with both bounding box and class probability assignments. Considering medical imaging, object detection can be used to simplify the clinical analysis process as it offers automated localization of areas of interest, decreases the level of human work, and enhances consistency in diagnoses (Ouadiay et al., 2018).

3.7.1.1 One-Stage vs Two-Stage Detectors

The detectors of objects are broadly categorized into two as follows:

i. **Two-Stage Detectors** : Two-stage detectors include R-CNN, Fast R-CNN, and Faster R-CNN where the initial phase of the model generates region proposals and the second stage for classification. They are very accurate and are mostly applied in applications that involve high accuracy in localization. They are however, slower in computation and not very appropriate in real time applications.

ii. **One-Stage Detectors :** Single-stage detectors such as YOLO and SSD, do not generate region proposals, and detect in one step. These are high-speed models that are competitive enough in terms of accuracy. They are best suited to real-time medical imaging processes that need a quick analysis (Olorunshola et al., 2023).

3.7.1.2 YOLO Family Overview

The YOLO (You Only Look Once) family represents a series of one-stage object detectors designed for real-time detection. YOLO has evolved through multiple versions, with each improving speed, accuracy, and architectural efficiency.**YOLOv1-v3** is a one-stage detection design with significant speed advantages. YOLOv4-v5 has improved feature extraction, training stability, and detection accuracy. YOLOv7 has optimized computational efficiency and enhanced model depth-width scaling. **YOLOv8** is the latest generation offering modular design, an advanced backbone, and improved detection heads. YOLO models are widely used in biomedical applications for their real-time performance and strong detection of small or irregular objects, such as follicles.

3.7.1.3 YOLOv8 Architecture

YOLO (You Only Look Once) family It is a family of single-stage detectors of objects that are capable of real-time detection. YOLO has had several releases with each generation achieving faster, more precise, and architecture-efficient designs.YOLOv1-v3 is a single-stage detector that has major speed gains. YOLOv4-v5 has a better feature extraction, stable training, and accuracy of detection. YOLOv7 has maximized the computational efficiency and the depth-width scaling of models. YOLOv8 has been the most recent generation that has been designable with a more complex backbone and detectable heads. YOLO models are commonly applicable in biomedical purposes due to their real-time capability as well as their ability to detect small or irregular objects, e.g. follicles, effectively.

3.7.1.4 Feature Aggregation (Neck) and Detection Head

The neck part determines the features at various scales using the backbone in order to provide the effective search of both small and large features.YOLOv8 realizes its features combination using PAN-FPN (Path Aggregation Network-Feature Pyramide Network), which combines the information of both low and high-resolution layers. This combination of features has been demonstrated to identify follicles of different sizes with this model which is critical in the PCOS ultrasound examination. The detection head provides three kinds of outputs, namely, bounding boxes, objectness score, and class probability prediction (Gan et al., 2025). In the anchor-free detection head of YOLOv8, the object centers and box sizes are directly forecasted, enhancing their accuracy and easing training. The process enhances identification of tiny and overlapping structures that are usually apparent in ultrasound images.

3.7.2 Theory of Bounding Box Regression

Bounding box regression is the process of learning how to compare the predicted bounding boxes and the real location of the objects. The goal is to reduce the variation of the predicted and actual box parameters, which are usually in the form of center coordinates (x, y) width (w) and height (h). Models are taught to refine predicted boxes by calculating offsets in respect to set grid cells or anchors. Regression enhances the detection strength especially in small objects in anchor-free models such as the YOLOv8 which directly predicts box boundaries on pixel-level features.

3.7.3 Loss Functions in Detection

Loss functions help to train detection models by penalizing wrong predictions. YOLOv8 has a series of following multiple loss components that are as follows:

(i) **Localization Loss:** It is the measure of the quality of the prediction of the bounding box against the ground truth. Geometric prediction penalty. The inaccurate geometry prediction is frequently penalized by metrics like IoU, GIoU, DIoU and CIoU.

(ii) **Objectness Loss:** It defines whether a box that is being predicted contains an object or not. This assists in the minimization of false positives and better scoring of confidence.

(iii) **Classification Loss:** This measures the loss in bad class prediction. In the case of multi-class entropy, Binary Cross-Entropy (BCE) is normally taken as the multi-class predictions of YOLOv8. An aggregate of these factors is the total detection loss, which makes sure that there is a compromise between accurate classification of object presence and the localization.

3.8 MULTI-SCALE FEATURE FUSION

Multi-scale feature fusion is a common feature in most deep learning models that are aimed at performing object detection and medical image analysis tasks. The model is more effective in extracting features by processing the information at varying levels of spatial scale, thus it is able to identify small features and large trends. Multi-scale fusion leads to an improvement in the detection of follicles of various sizes, and this is useful in the detection of PCOS in an ultrasound setting, to isolate the follicles among other ovarian structures.

3.8.1 Need for Multi-Scale Learning

Medical images show objects at different scales because imaging conditions, anatomical differences, and zoom levels create these variations. Detecting small, low-contrast structures is difficult for traditional convolutional neural networks because spatial information degrades with increasing network depth. The network achieves better results through multi-scale learning by combining information from different network layers. The model preserves both fine follicle details and complete ovarian shape information while maintaining stable performance across different scales. The multi-scale learning approach enables precise detection and segmentation of structures of varying sizes in ultrasound images.

3.8.2 Feature Pyramid Concept

One of the most popular ways of modeling more than one scale is the Feature Pyramid. It constructs a pyramid of characteristic maps of the decreasing resolution with the growth of semantic richness. The Feature Pyramid Network (FPN) is a combination of the following:

(i) **Bottom-up pathway**: Extraction of features with the help of the backbone network.
(ii) **Top-down connection**: Upsampling of high-level features.
(iii) **Lateral connections**: Fusion between level corresponding feature maps. The structure allows the network to have a high semantic meaning across the different scales thus making it detect small and big objects correctly.

FNPs are beneficial to the medical ultrasound imaging process to enhance the visibility of follicles and minimize erroneous interpretation of tissue patterns.

3.8.3 Attention-Guided Multi-Scale Fusion

Attention-guided fusion combines multi-scale features using spatial and channel attention approaches. Instead of treating all features equally, attention was given to the most informative features on each scale, and they were assigned higher weights during fusion. This approach enhances the model's ability to focus on clinically important regions, to suppress irrelevant or noisy information (e.g., speckle), and improve detection accuracy for small and overlapping structures. In PCOS images, attention-guided multi-scale fusion helps the model to emphasize significant follicular boundaries while reducing confusion caused by heterogeneous ovarian textures.

3.8.4 Mathematical Modeling

Multi-scale feature fusion can be expressed as a weighted combination of feature maps at different levels.

Given feature maps $F_1, F_2, \ldots, F_n$ from different scales, a generalized fusion operation can be modelled as:

$$F_{\text{fused}} = \sum_{i=1}^{n} w_i \cdot U(F_i) \tag{36}$$

where ,

- $\boldsymbol{F_i}$ is Feature map at scale *i*
- $\boldsymbol{U}(\cdot)$ is Up sampling or down sampling operator
- $\boldsymbol{w_i}$: Fusion weight for scale *i*, which may be learned through an attention mechanism.

If attention is used, the weights may be expressed as:

$$w_i = \text{softmax}(A(F_i)) \tag{37}$$

where, $\boldsymbol{A}(\cdot)$ is an attention function that computes importance scores based on spatial, channel, or self-attention mechanisms. This mathematical formulation ensures that the fused feature representation integrates both low-level spatial detail and high-level semantic understanding.

3.9 SQUEEZE-AND-EXCITATION (SE) BLOCKS

Squeeze-and-excitation blocks (SE) are an architectural building block which is used to increase the representational power of the coevolutionary neural network by explicitly modeling channel-wise dependencies. SE-Net presented SE blocks, which won the ILSVRC classification by the increase of both efficiency and accuracy without the significant increase of the complexity. The channels of the SE blocks accomplished rebalancing of response functions, enhancing the essential information and decreasing the helpless signals.

3.9.1 Channel Recalibration Concept

The traditional CNN applies convolutional filters to different channels to obtain features without having to take into account their interrelations with other channels. To overcome this limitation, the SE block recalibrates channels with global contextual information to find information on the importance weights of each channel.
The system is such that all channels must give equal value in the final predictions that the system will make. This system has two categories of channels where one channel is used to transmit non-vital data and another channel used to identify vital patterns of the ultrasound images. SE blocks allow the network to learn the features to concentrate on important features by dynamically modulating the channel response to select features better. The network is made more receptive of significant patterns within the entire process.

3.9.2 Squeeze Operation

The squeeze operation records the global spatial data and reduces it to a small-sized channel description. This is through performance of **Global Average Pooling (GAP)** to every feature map.

Mathematically, for a feature map $X \in \mathrm{R}^{H \times W \times C}$, the squeezed vector $z \in R^{C}$ is computed as:

$$z_c = \frac{1}{H \times W} \sum_{i=1}^{H} \sum_{j=1}^{W} X_c(i,j) \tag{38}$$

This turns each channel into one scalar value which is the total global significance of that channel. The step will allow the network to acquire international contextual information, which is also important in medical imaging activities where structural patterns can be extensive.

3.9.3 Excitation Operation

The squeezed vector is used to learn channel specific weights in the excitation operation using a small feed-forward gating network. This network consists of:

i. An r-dimensional dimensional reduction (FC) layer to model cross-channel interactions.
ii. A non-linear activation (ReLU). The other FC layer to dimensionality.
iii. A sigmoid-based activation in order to produce weights in the ranges of 0 to 1.

Mathematically:

$$\boldsymbol{s} = \sigma(\boldsymbol{W}_2\, \delta(\boldsymbol{W}_1 \boldsymbol{z})) \tag{39}$$

where ,

- $\boldsymbol{W}_1 \in \mathbf{R}^{\frac{C}{r} \times C}$
- $\boldsymbol{W}_2 \in \mathbf{R}^{C \times \frac{C}{r}}$

- $\boldsymbol{\delta}$ is **ReLU**, $\boldsymbol{\sigma}$is the sigmoid function
- $\boldsymbol{s} \in \mathbf{R}^{C}$is the channel attention vector.

These weights are then applied to the feature maps through channel-wise multiplication:

$$\boldsymbol{s} = \sigma\left(\boldsymbol{W}_2\, \delta(\boldsymbol{W}_1 \boldsymbol{z})\right) \tag{40}$$

$$\widetilde{\boldsymbol{X}}_c = \boldsymbol{s}_c \cdot \boldsymbol{X}_c \tag{41}$$

This selectively amplifies channels with strong discriminative power and suppresses weak or noisy channels.

3.9.4 Benefits of SE Blocks

SE blocks have several advantages, as follows:

i. **Improved Discrimination of features:** SE blocks are used to model interdependencies between channels to allow the network to learn and reinforce important features. It is crucial most in the ultrasound imaging, where one requires to identify fine boundaries, textures, and follicles correctly.
ii. **Parameters Efficiency:** The number of parameters added by them is very small (reduction ratio r). Nonetheless, they lead to the considerable accuracy improvements.
iii. **Better Gradient Flow**: Trained channels are also fixed to stabilize the training and cause a smoother gradient propagation.
iv. **Enhanced Performance on Tasks:** SE blocks always enhance classification, detection, segmentation and denoising task.

v. **Portability to Alternative Architectures:** They are usable in both shallow and deep networks without having to make any adjustments to the architecture in use. The CNN architectures are also integrated with the silicon in 3.9.5.

SE blocks are very modular and can be easily incorporated into the common convolutional layers. Under normal circumstances, the Squeeze-and-Excitation block follows the convolutional and batch normalization blocks and is immediately followed by the activation function.

Such popular integrations are type:

i. **SE-ResNet:** It incorporates the SE blocks within every residual block to strengthen skip-connected features.

ii. **SE-Inception:** This helps to improve the architecture of Inception by re-calibrating the multi-branch outputs.

iii. **SE-DenseNet:** Enhances feature reuse in a dense way by using channel-wise attention. Lightweight Models (MobileNet, ShuffleNet): SE blocks also can be used to enhance the performance of mobile models with few computational costs.

Squeeze-and-excited (SE) blocks regularly find applications in U-Net, ResNet, and EfficientNet architectures in the field of medical imaging. This integration increases the feature localization, refines boundary identification and increases noise-resistance, particularly in ultrasound images, where speckle noise and low contrast is a challenge.

4.0 RESIDUAL NETWORKS (RESNET)

One of the most significant improvements to deep learning architectures has been Residual Networks (ResNets), which allow it to train an extremely deep convolutional neural network without either vanishing gradients or a drop in performance. Introduced by He et al. in 2015, ResNet added residual learning and skip connections to enable networks with hundreds of layers to easily converge and also achieve state-of-the-art accuracy at all vision tasks.

4.0.1 Limitations of Deep CNNs

Convolutional neural networks have a number of issues with training as they get deeper:

i. **Vanishing and Exploding Gradients:** The gradients either diminish or become uncontrollable during the process of backpropagation by passing through several layers and updating early layers becomes a challenge. This makes very deep architecture training impossible.

ii. **Degradation Problem:** The accuracy of a plain CNN sometimes does not increase with the addition of more layers. After a point of sufficient depth, performance levels off and after that, it begins to decrease not due to overfitting but due to optimization problems.

iii. **Problem of propagating features**: Deep networks are also poor at propagating low-level features (edges, textures) to the higher levels leading to the loss of valuable information.

iv. **Slow Convergence**: Sluggish plain networks approach convergence slowly and need cautious strategies of initializing them. ResNet has conquered these shortcomings by allowing identity-mapping shortcuts which preserve the network gradient flow and do not miss important information.

4.0.2 Skip Connections

The invention of ResNet is the so-called shortcut connections, or more precisely, skip connections. ResNet does not learn a direct mapping between the input x and the output H(x), but a residual function:

$$F(x) = H(x) - x \Rightarrow H(x) = F(x) + x \tag{42}$$

where,

- $x$is the input to the block
- $F(x)$are the outputs of stacked convolution layers and the identity mapping
- $x$is added directly to the transformed features

There are advantages of skip connections as follows:

i. Gradient flow Gradient flow will not vanish.

ii. Training of very deep networks possible.

iii. This enables the model to learn the changes in identity transformation.

iv. Enhance optimization comfort and speed of convergence.

v. Support feature Reuse between layers.

In this way, deep networks can be made to act like shallow network ensembles with skip connections. Thus, skip connections allow deep networks to behave more like ensembles of shallower networks.

4.0.3 Residual Block Structure

The following are the constituents of a residual block:

i. **Convolutional layers:** There are typically two or three convolution layers (3x3) or (1x1) that are stacked.

ii. **BN:** Stable training and accelerated convergence.

iii. **ReLU Activation:** Adds non-linearity in between convolutions.

iv. **Identity (Skip) Connection:** This connection sums the input of the elements of the convolution layers to the result.

v. **Basic Residual Block (ResNet18/34):** It consists of 2x3x3 convolution layers.

vi. **Bottleneck Residual Block (ResNet50/101/152):** It consists of three layers viz. 1x1 convolution (dimension reduction), 3x3 convolution (feature extraction) and 1x1 convolution (dimension restoration).

Mathematically:

$$\boldsymbol{y} = \boldsymbol{F}(\boldsymbol{x}, \boldsymbol{W}) + \boldsymbol{x} \tag{43}$$

where,

- ***W*** represents the block's weights.

This bottleneck design reduces computational cost and enables deeper architectures without incurring high memory costs.

4.0.4 ResNet50 Architecture

ResNet50 is powerful and efficient in that it has 50 layers containing bottleneck residual blocks. ResNet50 is designed as a network with 7x7 convolution layer of 64 filters and then with max pooling then 4 sequential stages-Conv2x with 3 bottlenecks producing 256 channels, Conv3x with 4 bottlenecks producing 512 channels, Conv4x with 6 bottlenecks producing 1024 channels and Conv5x with 3 bottlenecks producing 2048 channels after which global average pooling and a fully connected layer (originally optimized to 1000 ImageNet classes

4.0.5 Benefits of Medical Imaging :

The ResNet50 and its variants have been the benchmark models of medical image analysis because they are robust and have the ability to extract deep features.

i. **Stability to Noise and Artifacts:** Skip connections are designed to preserve low-level textures and can therefore enable the network to be robust to speckle noise in ultrasound images.

ii. **Successful Feature Propagation:** Residual learning will guarantee that significant spatial and structural data will be propagated across the layers which will help in identifying a small lesion, follicles, cysts or boundaries.

iii. **Excellent in Transfer Learning:** ImageNet pretrained models are able to be adapted to medical datasets that tend to be small and imbalanced.

iv. **Enhanced Gradient Stability:** This architecture also trains well in situations when only limited data is available, which is typical in clinical research.

v. **High Performance in Tasks:** ResNet is applicable in PCOS follicle detection, tumor classification, organ segmentation, disease prediction, and medical image denoising and reconstruction.

Interoperability with Modern Modules ResNet is compatible with attention modules (SE, CBAM, Transformer), multi-scale feature extractors, detection models (YOLO, Faster R-CNN), and explainable AI models (Grad-CAM, Score-CAM). ResNet50 has these strengths that enable it to be a suitable deep learning-based backbone in diagnostic imaging tasks.

4.1 EXPLAINABLE AI TECHNIQUES (XAI)

Explainable Artificial Intelligence (XAI) is a collection of techniques created to render the choices of deep learning models visible, comprehensible, and decipherable to human specialists. In medical imaging, the issue of interpretability is not discretionary; medical diagnoses, which directly influence the outcome of the patients, are involved. XAI closes the structure between high-performing black-box models and clinical trust and provides visual and mathematical explanations of model predictions.

4.1.1 Need for Interpretability in Medical AI

Deep learning models, especially CNNs in the field of medical image diagnosis, are usually black boxes. This is not very transparent, which presents a number of problems:

i. **Clinical Trust and Acceptance:** Radiologists and clinicians need clear grounds on the basis of automated predictions. XAI identifies the areas that affect the decision of the model in detail, which enhances its confidence and adoption.

ii. **Regulatory and Ethical Conditions:** Medical AI systems will have to be able to meet the standards of explainability established by regulatory authorities (e.g., FDA, EU AI Act). Accountability and safety are guaranteed through explainability.

iii. **Error Analysis and Debugging:** XAI assists the researcher in determining whether the model is targeting the right anatomical areas or is being misguided by artifacts, noise, and irrelevant structures.

iv. **Detection and Reduction of bias:** Interpretability can be used to detect any bias or imbalance of the data by displaying which features are used by the model.

v. **Clinical Collaboration:** Visualization-based explanations can help improve the communication between AI researchers and clinicians to improve model refinement.

Hence, XAI plays a crucial role in improving performance, reliability, and clinical usefulness in addition to transparency.

4.1.2 Class Activation Mapping (CAM)

Class Activation Mapping (CAM) is one of the earliest interpretability techniques for CNNs. CAM identifies the **discriminative image regions** that contribute to a model's prediction. **Class Activation Mapping (CAM)** works by using a CNN architecture that includes convolutional layers to extract spatial features, a Global Average Pooling

(GAP) layer to convert each feature map into a single representative value, and a fully connected classification layer whose learned weights are used to compute a weighted combination of the final convolutional feature maps, producing a heatmap that highlights the region's most responsible for the model's prediction. For a predicted class c, CAM computes a weighted sum of the activation maps from the last convolutional layer.

Mathematically:

$$\boldsymbol{M_c(x,y)} = \sum_{k} \boldsymbol{w_k^c} \cdot \boldsymbol{A_k(x,y)} \tag{44}$$

where ,

- $\boldsymbol{A_k(x,y)}$ is the activation map of the channel k,
- $\boldsymbol{w_k^c}$ is Weight for class $c$associated with the channel k and
- $\boldsymbol{M_c(x,y)}$ The heatmap highlights important regions.

CAM has notable limitations: it works only with specific CNN architectures that include a Global Average Pooling layer, meaning it cannot be directly applied to standard classification or detection models such as ResNet or YOLO without architectural modifications. These constraints motivated the development of more general and flexible explainability methods, such as **Grad-CAM.**

4.1.3 Gradient-Weighted CAM (Grad-CAM).

Grad-CAM overcomes the structural limitations of CAM. It can be applied to any CNN, including ResNet, DenseNet, VGG, YOLO detectors, and Segmentation networks. Grad-CAM generates a class-specific localization map by using gradients flowing into the last convolutional layer. Grad-CAM Works in the following steps:

Step 1: Compute gradients of the class score y^c with respect to the feature maps A_k:

$$\frac{\partial y^c}{\partial A_k} \tag{45}$$

Step 2: Global average pool the gradients to obtain importance weights:

$$\alpha_k^c = \frac{1}{Z}\sum_i \sum_j \frac{\partial y^c}{\partial A_k(i,j)} \tag{46}$$

Step 3: Generate the weighted sum of the feature maps:

$$L^c_{Grad\text{-}CAM} = ReLU\left(\sum_k \alpha_k^c A_k\right) \tag{47}$$

The ReLU ensures only positive influences are visualized.

Grad-CAM offers several advantages: it is model-agnostic across CNN-based architectures, provides coarse yet meaningful localization of important image regions, requires no architectural modifications, and is highly effective across classification, detection, and medical imaging tasks.

4.1.4 Mathematical Derivations

Below is a compact derivation of Grad-CAM used in a research thesis.

1. Class Score Function

For class c, the model outputs a score:

$$y^c = f(A_1, A_2, \dots, A_K) \tag{48}$$

2. Gradient Computation

We compute gradients of the class score with respect to activation maps:

$$\frac{\partial y^c}{\partial A_k(i,j)} \tag{49}$$

3. Importance Weights

The gradients are averaged spatially:

$$\alpha_k^c = \frac{1}{Z}\sum_{i=1}^{H}\sum_{j=1}^{W}\frac{\partial y^c}{\partial A_k(i,j)} \tag{50}$$

4. Heatmap Construction

The localization map is created using:

$$L_c(i,j) = ReLU\left(\sum_{k=1}^{K}\alpha_k^c A_k(i,j)\right) \tag{51}$$

5. Normalization

The heatmap is normalized:

$$L_c' = \frac{L_c - min(L_c)}{max(L_c) - min(L_c)} \tag{52}$$

This generates a clinically interpretable heatmap highlighting the region's most relevant to the model's decision.

4.1.5 Visualization and Clinical Relevance

The use of AI models to interpret visualizations of medical imaging hugely depends on XAI visualizations.

i. **Findings Key Pathological Regions:** Grad-CAM heatmaps show the specific parts of the image affecting the model-e.g. large follicles, cyst edges or ovarian folklore in PCOS ultrasound.

ii. **Helping Clinical Decision-Making:** The clinicians would be able to confirm whether the attention of the model is consistent with the existing anatomical or pathological indicators.

iii. **Identifying Model Failures:** Heatmaps are used to identify instances of the model being concentrated on irrelevant structures, bright artifacts, or noise that are used to improve the system. Improving Training and Data Quality A visual explanation facilitates the process of dataset curation, augmentation, and model redesign.

iv. **Enhancing Trust, Transparency, and Adoption:** XAI will help fill the gap between AI research and clinical practice and will raise the level of acceptance in hospitals and diagnostic centers.

v. **Applicable to Explainable Diagnostics and Regulatory Approval:** Explanations can help justify the use of AI and its regulation by law.

4.2 EVALUATION METRICS

The use of evaluation metrics is very important in measuring the performance of deep learning models developed to perform medical imaging tasks. To measure accuracy, robustness, and reliability, different quantitative values are applied, depending on the task (denoising, classification, or detection). This part presents frequently employed measurements and clarifies the mathematical value of these measurements, particularly regarding ultrasound-based PCOS detection and its uses.

4.2.1 Denoising Metrics

The denoising metrics of an algorithm evaluate how well the algorithm removes noise in an image whilst maintaining important structural details.

4.2.1.1 Peak Signal-to-Noise Ratio (PSNR)

Peak Signal-to-Noise Ratio (PSNR) measures the ratio between the maximum possible pixel intensity and the error introduced by the denoising algorithm.

It is given by:

$$\text{PSNR} = 10 \log_{10}\left(\frac{MAX^2}{MSE}\right) \tag{53}$$

where:

$$MSE = \frac{1}{HW}\sum_{i=1}^{H} \sum_{j=1}^{W} (I(i,j) - \hat{I}(i,j))^2 \tag{54}$$

where,

- I: Original image
- $\hat{I}$: Denoised image
- MAX: Maximum pixel value

Interpretation:

- Higher PSNR indicates better denoising quality.
- Commonly used for ultrasound, MRI, CT, and X-ray restoration.

4.2.1.2 Structural Similarity Index (SSIM)

Structural Similarity Index (SSIM) evaluates the perceptual similarity between the original and denoised image by considering luminance, contrast, and structural information.

$$SSIM(x,y) = \frac{(2\mu_x\mu_y + C_1)(2\sigma_{xy} + C_2)}{(\mu_x^2 + \mu_y^2 + C_1)(\sigma_x^2 + \sigma_y^2 + C_2)} \tag{55}$$

where,

- μ_x, μ_y: Mean intensities
- σ_x^2, σ_y^2: Variances
- σ_{xy}: Covariance
- C_1, C_2: Stability constants

Interpretation:

- SSIM ranges from -1 to 1
- 1 indicates perfect structural similarity
- Better suited for medical imaging than PSNR because it captures perceptual quality and anatomical fidelity

4.2.2 Classification Metrics

Classification metrics are used to evaluate models that categorize images into different classes (e.g., PCOS vs normal ovary).

These metrics are based on four fundamental quantities:

- **TP** (True Positive)
- **TN** (True Negative)
- **FP** (False Positive)
- **FN** (False Negative)

4.2.2.1 Accuracy

Measures the overall correctness of the model.

$$Accuracy = \frac{TP + TN}{TP + TN + FP + FN} \tag{56}$$

Use: Good for balanced datasets, but misleading when classes are imbalanced.

4.2.2.2 Precision

Indicates how many of the predicted positive cases are truly positive.

$$Precision = \frac{TP}{TP + FP} \tag{57}$$

Use: Important in medical diagnosis to reduce false alarms.

4.2.2.3 Recall

Also called sensitivity or true positive rate.

$$Recall = \frac{TP}{TP + FN} \tag{58}$$

Use: Critical for medical applications because missing a disease case is more dangerous than a false positive.

4.2.2.4 F1-Score

Harmonic mean of precision and recall:

$$F1 = 2 \times \frac{Precision \cdot Recall}{Precision + Recall} \tag{59}$$

Use: Best metric when classes are imbalanced.

4.2.2.5 ROC-AUC

The Receiver Operating Characteristic - Area Under Curve (ROC-AUC) measures the trade-off between sensitivity and specificity across thresholds.

- AUC ranges from 0 to 1

- Higher AUC indicates better model separability

Use: Widely used in medical AI to assess reliability across classification thresholds.

4.2.3 Detection Metrics

Detection metrics are used for object detection tasks such as identifying and localizing follicles or cysts in ultrasound images.

4.2.3.1 Intersection over Union (IoU)

IoU measures the overlap between the predicted bounding box and the ground truth box.

$$IoU = \frac{Area(B_{pred} \cap B_{gt})}{Area(B_{pred} \cup B_{gt})} \tag{60}$$

Interpretation:

- IoU ≥ 0.5 is typically considered a correct detection (PASCAL VOC)
- Higher IoU indicates better localization accuracy

4.2.3.2 Mean Average Precision (mAP)

mAP is the most widely used metric for object detection models such as YOLO, Faster R-CNN, and SSD.

Steps:

1. Compute precision-recall curve for each class
2. Calculate Average Precision (AP)
3. Take the mean of AP across all classes:

$$mAP = \frac{1}{N}\sum_{i=1}^{N} AP_i \tag{61}$$

Interpretation:

- Higher mAP means better detection performance
- mAP@50: IoU threshold = 0.50
- mAP@50–95: averaged across IoU thresholds 0.50 to 0.95

In medical imaging, mAP indicates how accurately structures are detected and localized.

4.3. CHAPTER SUMMARY

This chapter provided an overview of the main ideas of artificial intelligence applications in medical image analysis, namely, deep learning in PCOS detection based on ultrasound. The study commenced with simple approaches as autoencoders and attention mechanisms, the properties of speckle noise, and advanced approaches to image denoising, object detection, multi-scale features combination, Squeeze-and-Excitation blocks, and Residual Networks (ResNet).

The explanations of CAM and Grad-CAM explainable AI methods showed that model interpretability is a very important consideration in clinical settings. To develop standardized criteria of performance evaluation, the paper introduced evaluation measures of denoising, classification, and detection.

These ideas provide the theoretical framework of the development of reliable AI systems in medical imaging that will underpin the methodological and experimental work that follows.

CHAPTER-4

METHODOLOGY

4.1 INTRODUCTION

This study aims to develop an optimized deep learning technique to facilitate the early detection of PCOS using ovarian ultrasound data in a reliable, accurate, and computationally efficient manner. Particularly, a few deep learning methods will be examined and discussed in the context of the PCOS detection of ultrasound images. Taking into account the character of the issue and the nature of the information, a quantitative and experimental method was selected, which employed state-of-the-art deep learning and medical image analysis methods. This study leveraged deep learning, particularly the attention mechanism within autoencoders, to enhance ultrasound image quality and support more accurate and reliable PCOS detection, aligning with the broader goals of digital health innovation and SDGs 3 and 9. The strategy relies much on the gathering and distribution of good-quality ultrasound images, including those of people with and without PCOS. Preprocessing of all input images is required to put deep learning models into a standardized and trained form. Here, overfitting reduction and model robustness are enhanced with the use of cropping, resizing, and augmentation. As a rule, to enhance the visualization of the structure of cyst and follicle patterns in the ovary, domain-specific preprocessing steps are performed. Once the data is prepared, different deep learning constructions are used, the newest transfer learning models, and the traditional CNN models. Subsequently, accuracy, precision, recall, F1-score, and area under ROC curve (AUC) are evaluated as a performance criterion of each model that has been trained, validated and tested on a chosen data sets after completion. These data confirm the clinical relevance and diagnostic issue of the model. To create reproducible and reliable results, cross-validation methods, statistical tests, as well as performance comparison against known methods also become part of the methodology. The experimental design has been designed in such a way that it allows a remarkable and breakthrough innovation of the proposed optimized models against already existing baseline techniques, and validates their effectiveness in real-world diagnostic setups. Apart from this, special attention is kept in terms of the model's interpretability, by using tools like Grad-CAM to represent feature activations and validation of the models that focus upon medically relevant regions of the image.

4.2 DATA COLLECTION

Data collection is a crucial first step in any study. Publicly available and medically verified ultrasound images of ovaries have been used to develop optimized deep learning techniques for the detection of PCOS. Below the table 4.1 and 4.2 gives summary of the datasets used throughout the research work done for developing a noise reduction model and a diagnostic model, which is as follows:

Table 4.1 Dataset Used for Noise Reduction Model

Parameter	Description
Dataset Type	Publicly available PCOS ultrasound image dataset
Total Images	3,856 images
Training Images	2,685 images
Testing Images	671 images
Image Format	RGB ultrasound images
Image Size	128 × 128 × 3 pixels
Noise Simulation	Synthetic speckle noise added with variance levels 0.5, 0.02, and 0.001
Purpose	To train and evaluate the Multi-Level Attention Autoencoder (AAE) for noise reduction

Evaluation Metrics	PSNR (Peak Signal-to-Noise Ratio) and SSIM (Structural Similarity Index Measure)

Table 4.2: Dataset used for Developing Diagnostic Model

Parameter	Kaggle PCOS Dataset
Source	Public dataset from Kaggle (*PCOS Detection Using Ultrasound Images*, n.d.)
Total Images	3,856 (approx.)
Training Images	1,932
Testing Images	1,924
Class Distribution	781 PCOS-positive, 1,143 normal
Annotation	Manual labelling by domain experts
Image Size	128 × 128 × 3 pixels
Data Augmentation	Rotation, zooming, horizontal/vertical flip, shearing
Purpose	For training YOLOv8-based follicle detection and SE-ResNet50 classification model
Evaluation Metrics	Accuracy, Precision, Recall, F1-Score, ROC-AUC, mAP
Remarks	Dataset re-partitioned to ensure fair training and testing

4.3 SYSTEM SPECIFICATIONS

The hardware and software prerequisites for this research are described in Tables 4.3 and 4.4, respectively.

4.3.1 HARDWARE SPECIFICATION:

The hardware environment used for model training and testing in this research is summarized as follows:

Table 4.3 Hardware Specification

S.No.	Component	Specification
1.	CPU Processor	Intel(R) Core(TM) i7-11700, 2.50 GHz
2.	Graphics Processing Unit	NVIDIA GeForce RTX 3060
3.	GPU Memory	6 GB
4.	System Memory	32 GB
5.	Storage	1 TB SSD
6.	Operating System	Windows 11 (64-bit)
7.	Display Resolution	1920 × 1080 pixels

4.3.2 SOFTWARE SPECIFICATIONS

The software environment used for model training and testing in this research is summarized as follows:

Table 4.4 Software Specifications

S.No.	Software/Tool	Version/Description
1.	Operating System	Windows 11(64-bit)
2.	Programming Language	Python 3.10
3.	Deep Learning Frameworks	TensorFlow and Keras for AAE; PyTorch for YOLOv8 and SE-ResNet50
4.	Supporting Libraries	NumPy, Pandas, OpenCV, Scikit-learn, Matplotlib

5.	Annotation Tool	Roboflow and Labelling (for bounding box generation)
6.	Visualization Tools	Tensor Board and Grad-CAM
7.	Optimization Algorithm	Adam Optimizer
8.	Evaluation Metrics	PSNR, SSIM, Accuracy, Precision, Recall, F1-Score, and mAP

4.4 METHODOLOGY FOR OBJECTIVE 1:

To Collect Data and Detect Polycystic Ovarian Syndrome through Ultrasound Images using Deep Learning Technique.

4.4.1 Introduction

The first objective of this research is to systematically collect, prepare, and use ultrasound images to detect Polycystic Ovary Syndrome (PCOS) using deep learning techniques. The primary non-invasive diagnostic modality for PCOS is Ultrasound imaging, which can visualize ovarian morphology; typical findings include multiple peripheral microfollicles, increased ovarian volume, and increased stromal echogenicity. These morphological characteristics are important for differentiating between polycystic ovaries and normal ovaries and thus lay the foundation for automated, computer-aided detection systems.

Primarily for PCOS analysis and diagnosis, the dataset is taken from Kaggle(*PCOS Detection Using Ultrasound Images*, n.d.) containing 3,856 ultrasound images collected for PCOS analysis and diagnosis. Initially, 1,932 images were used for training data, and 1,924 for testing data. Later, because of significant overlap between the original training and testing datasets, the original test set was discarded, and the entire dataset was reorganized to create new, non-overlapping training and testing partitions.

The dataset contains two categories: INFECTED, with 781 images of cystic ovaries, and NOT INFECTED, with 1,143 images of normal ovaries. Fig. 4.1 represents the infected and non-infected classes of ultrasound images. The labelling of infected and non-infected indicates individuals diagnosed with PCOS and those without the condition, respectively, enabling automated, accurate classification in real-time medical systems.

To improve the dataset, a later another set of datasets was taken from the **PCOSGen** dataset (*PCOSGen-Train Dataset*, n.d.), compiled from multiple online sources. This dataset contains 1,468 images of infected ovaries and 3,200 images of noninfected ovaries. Here, all samples were annotated by a qualified gynaecologist based in New Delhi. Later, the dataset was split into training and testing subsets to support model development and evaluation.

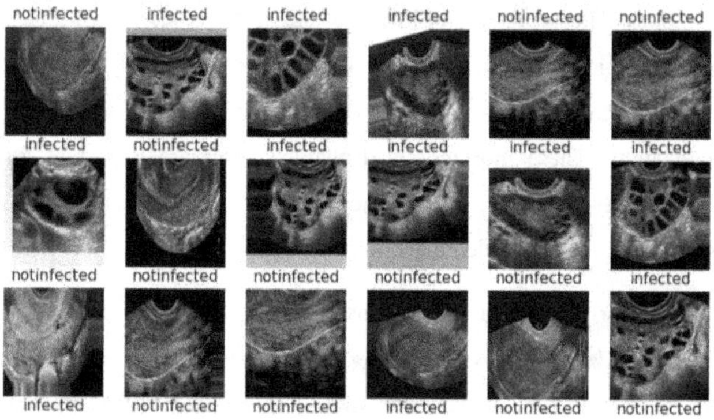

Fig. 4.1 Different sample images from both classes(infected and non-infected)

4.4.2 Preprocessing of the dataset

To ensure consistency and improve model performance, all ultrasound images underwent a standardized preprocessing pipeline. At this stage, the ultrasound images are first normalized by scaling pixel intensity values to the range 0 to 1. In order to reduce distortion a median filter is used that is known to be an effective filter of removing speckle noise in ultrasound images (Pandey et al., 2025a). The filter identifies the value of a given pixel and replaces the pixel value with the median of the given pixels around the pixel to decrease noise without distorting important image details. Finally, in order to standardize images with different size, we down-sample the images to 128x128x3. Ultrasound images are also prone to speckle noise and other artifacts in the given datasets; a noise reduction process was carried out using the median filtering and adaptive histogram equalization. The process enhances contrast and brings out the structures of the ovarian structures and pulls out the unwanted background noise. To make it even better, the images could also be cropped in case of highlighting of ovarian regions of interest (ROI) which made the model concentrate on the relevant anatomic features, and extraneous tissue was minimized.

4.4.3 Data Augmentation

In order to enhance the variety of training data and deter overfitting, a number of augmentation methods were utilized on the training images. It is an essential process regarding the case of computer vision which helps to expand the range of the dataset, as well as the variety, to help the models in generalizations and work properly in real life (Perez & Wang, 2017). In this research, zooming, rotation, flipping, and sharing augmentations were performed. These image alterations replicated real-life situations in which an object's position and orientation can change, producing numerous additional images that modify the originals (Pandey et al., 2025a). This has the advantage of reducing the risk of overfitting of the data set as well as making the model focus on different attributes, which enhance credible performance of different input data. Fig. 4.2 illustrates the various augmentation techniques applied to the images.

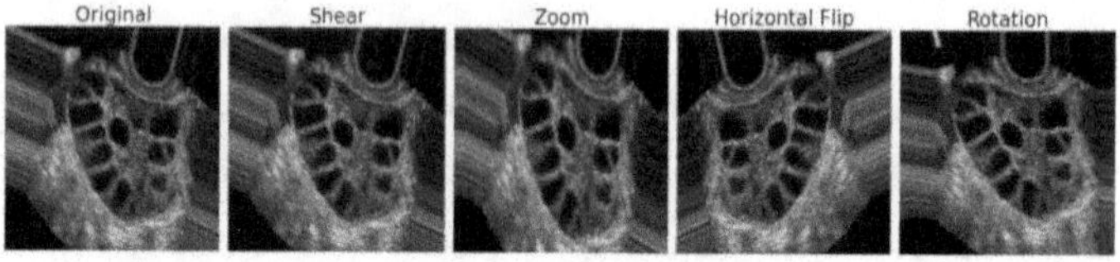

Fig. 4.2 : Various augmentation techniques applied on original images.

4.4.4 Follicle detection

Before performing the classification task, image detection in the polycystic ovary syndrome (PCOS) diagnosis domain is crucial. Follicles in the ovaries are perhaps one of the most significant grounds for diagnosing PCOS. Certainly, definite identification of these follicles in ultrasound images is critical for the identification of ROIs, which are very pertinent to abnormal ovarian morphology. In this research, to recognize follicles in ultrasound images, YOLOv8 (You Only Look Once Version 8) with the Attention-Guided Multi-Scale Feature Fusion (AGMSFF) module is used. This modification is making it easier for the model to distinguish among different follicle sizes in ultrasound images and to capture fine-grained details (Pandey et al., 2025a). The AGMSFF is introduced and integrated into the YOLOv8 architecture as a feature extractor and fusion model. It uses an Attention Mechanism alongside Multi-Scale Feature Fusion to fine-tune the predictions. The attention mechanism learns weights across the spatial and channel dimensions; the follicle boundaries are noteworthy, and negations are applied to unimportant parts. Mathematically, the attention mechanism can be expressed as:

$$\boldsymbol{F\_att = \sigma(W\_s \cdot GAP(F) \odot F} \tag{62}$$

Where F is the input feature map, σ denotes the sigmoid activation, W_s represents learnable parameters, and $GAP(F)(\cdot)$ is the global average pooling operation. The achieved attention-focused feature map F_{att} increases follicle-like regions determination. Multi-scale feature fusion is the method of integrating features achieved on different layers of the model such that the detection head may identify follicles of different sizes. Given feature maps F_1, F_2, F_3 from different scales, the fusion is performed as:

$$\boldsymbol{F_{fused} = F_1 + Up(F_2) + Up\big(Up(F_3)\big)} \tag{63}$$

where ,

$\boldsymbol{Up}(\cdot)$ represents up-sampling so as to align space. This multi-scale combining is not only to maintain fine details on a model but also a lot of contextual information which is critical in identifying small, irregularly shaped follicles. The enhanced YOLOv8 which is combined with AGMSFF processes ultrasound images to achieve follicles or bounding boxes. Every bounding box is coupled with both the confidence score S_c and a class label C, calculated as:

$$\boldsymbol{S_c = \sigma\big(W_c \cdot F_{fused}\big)} \tag{64}$$

where ,

W_c are classification weights. The output of this detection is further fed to the classification model. By incorporating this it enhances the detection performance for follicles identification.

4.5 METHODOLOGY FOR OBJECTIVE 2:

To develop a new filtering technique for the identification of follicles and reduction of speckle noise .

4.5.1. Introduction

Objective 2 is achieved by developing a new filtering technique for identifying follicles and speckle noise in ultrasound images. In modern diagnostics, medical imaging is crucial, particularly for conditions like polycystic ovary syndrome(PCOS), which can be diagnosed non-invasively using imaging modalities such as ultrasound. The problem, however, is that ultrasound imaging is notoriously susceptible to various types of noise, including speckle noise, which impedes diagnostic accuracy and degrades image quality. To mimic real-world imperfections and improve the model's resilience, synthetic speckle noise was added to the original ultrasound image dataset. In order to generate different noise intensities, speckle noise, a granular noise frequently seen in medical ultrasound imaging, was added at different variance levels. In digital image processing, the presence of unwanted variations in brightness or color information within an image. It's a kind of anomaly that obscures and distorts the original image data, making it difficult to analyze, interpret, and process, and negatively impacting the model's performance. Image noise is a random variation in brightness or color that manifests as a grainy, mottled, or snowy texture. Hence, we can say that noise is a biggest barrier in image classification because it reduces image quality making images looks look grainy, fuzzy, or less clear, difficulty in analysis i.e. it can interfere with the accuracy of tasks like object recognition, edge detection, and segmentation, which rely on precise pixel values and patterns and In sensitive fields like medical imaging or surveillance, noise can lead to misinterpretations or missed details, potentially impacting critical decisions i.e. leads to data misinterpretation. In lieu of further elaboration, let's explore type of noise that are described below. Generally, they fall into one of three categories :

i. **Gaussian Noise:**

Gaussian noise, commonly referred to as the Gaussian distribution, is a statistical noise with a probability density function equal to the normal distribution. This noise is produced by adding a random Gaussian function to the Image function. Because it occurs in amplifiers or detectors, it is also known as electronic noise.

ii. **Impulse Noise:**

Impulse Function: Impulse functions in the discrete world at a single point with a value of 1, and an idealized function with unit area is called an impulse function in the continuous world. Impulse noises come in three varieties. Pepper noise, salt noise, and pepper-and-salt noise.

a. ***Salt Noise:*** The inclusion of random bright pixels (with a 255-pixel value) throughout an image result in the addition of salt noise.
b. ***Pepper Noise:*** Random dark (with a 0-pixel value) is incorporated into an image to create salt noise.
c. ***Salt and Pepper Noise:*** Salt and Pepper noise is introduced to an image by introducing random bright (255-pixel value) and random dark (0-pixel value) elements throughout the image. This model is also referred to as data drop noise because it statistically reduces the original data values.

iii. Poisson Noise:

The statistical nature of electromagnetic radiation, including gamma rays, visible light, and X-rays, is the reason for the appearance of this noise. The number of photons emitted per unit time by the X-ray and gamma-ray sources. In medical X-ray and gamma-ray imaging systems, these particles are injected into the patient's body from their source. The photons from these sources are fluctuating at an unpredictable rate. The image obtained exhibits spatial and temporal irregularities. This noise is also called shot noise or quantum (photon) noise.

iv. Speckle Noise

Speckle noise during image reconstruction is one of the major issues in optical and digital holography. Speckle is noise that is granular and is inherent in images and reduces their quality. The speckle noise may be formed by multiplying random pixel values by the different pixels of an image. This is an issue that needs to come up with the strong image denoising methods to enhance image fidelity. The block diagram of the proposed denoised model appears in the block diagram in the below Fig. 4.3. Here, the preprocessing of the ultrasound images into uniformity is done initially and the speckle noise is added with different levels (0.001, 0.02 and 0.5) to evaluate the performance of the proposed method. The proposed denoising model is then fed with the noisy image. The proposed method retains relevant data to make a correct diagnosis because it produces a denoised image with less speckle noise. The attention mechanism presented in the block allows the model to highlight the main features, which boosts the denoising capability of the model in various degrees of noise. The following subsections address these steps.

4.5.2 Dataset description and noise addition

A publicly accessible dataset of ultrasound images associated with PCOS was used in this paper. The dataset includes 3,856 samples in total, each representing ultrasound images used for PCOS analysis and diagnosis. These photos provide vital visual information that helps detect cysts and other anomalies associated with illness. Machine learning and image processing tasks benefit greatly from the dataset's diversity, which includes a wide range of patient profiles and variations in PCOS manifestation.

Although the original ultrasound image dataset is clean, synthetic speckle noise was added in this study to mimic real-world imperfections and improve the model's resilience. Different noise intensities were produced by adding speckle noise, a granular noise commonly observed in medical ultrasound imaging, at varying levels of variance. For the suggested model to successfully remove noise from the photos, this step was essential for training. Applying the model to real-world noisy ultrasound images improved its generalization because it was exposed to a wide range of scenarios through simulated noise at varying intensities. A mathematical representation of the addition of speckle noise to a clear ultrasound image X is as follows:

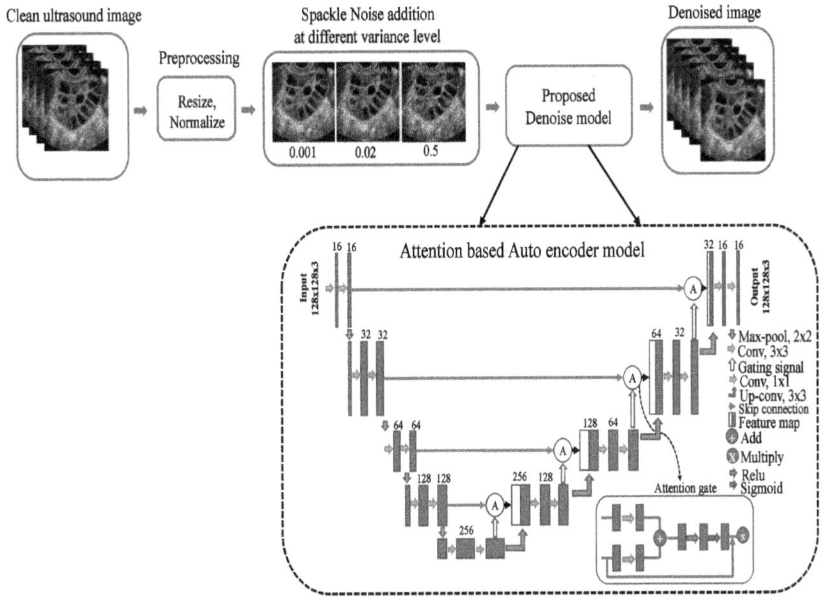

Fig. 4.3: Block Diagram of Proposed Denoise Method (Pandey et al., 2025b)

$$X_{noisy} = X + X \odot N \tag{65}$$

where X_{noisy} is the noisy image, X is the clean image, $N \sim N(0, \sigma^2)$ is the noise matrix sampled from a Gaussian distribution with mean 0 and σ^2 , and $\odot$ represents element-wise multiplication. The variance σ^2 is varied to simulate different levels of noise intensity, enabling the model to handle diverse noise conditions. Fig. 4.4 below illustrates a clean ultrasound image alongside versions with varying levels of added noise.

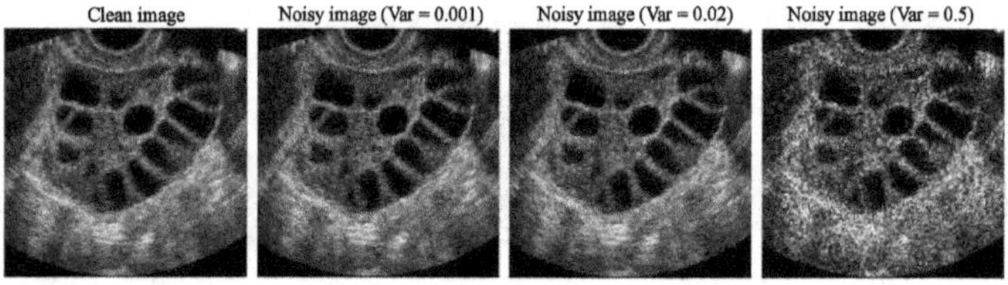

Fig. 4.4 : Clean ultrasound with noise image with varying levels of variance

4.5.3 Pre-processing

In this, various preprocessing techniques are employed to enhance the image quality before inputting it into the proposed method. As image sizes vary, we need to set a fixed size (128 x 128 x 3) for all images. To bring all image values into certain ranges, we used normalization techniques. Also used image smoothing to remove small artifacts while maintaining important features to improve performance. These processes maximize the output of the deep learning model by improving the accuracy and reliability of the input data.

4.5.4 Filtering method

As a filtering method, we used attention-based autoencoder (AAE) to adequately remove noise in the ultrasound images. Autoencoders are primarily divided into two components, an encoder, which takes the input image and translates it into a low-dimensional latent space, and a decoder that recovers the image based on the latent representation. In this study, we explained this architecture by incorporating an attention mechanism that enables the model to emphasize on the important features of the image to be classified thus enhancing the performance of the noise-removal. The mechanism of attention helps to enhance the effectiveness of the proposed attention-based autoencoder (AAE) through the selective focus on the salient areas of the image and noise reduction. Traditional autoencoders encode the input into a latent representation and reconstruct the image; they can often fail to differentiate important structures (e.g., ovarian cysts) and random noise patterns (e.g., speckle noise). An attention gate network is integrated to address this issue, dynamically modifying the feature representation by emphasizing relevant information and down weighting less significant areas.

For a given image the mathematically represented as shown below

$X_{noisy} \in R^{hxw}$	(66)

where h and w represent the height and width of the noisy image,

the encoder function $f_{encoder}(\cdot)$ projects X_{noisy} into a latent space $Z \in \mathbb{R}^{h'xw'xd}$,

where the number of channels represented by d, and h', w' are the dimensions of the compressed representation.

This can be represented as:

$$Z = f_{encoder}(X_{noisy}) \tag{67}$$

Next, the attention mechanism computes an attention map $A \in \mathbb{R}^{h'xw'xd}$, which assigns weights to different regions of the latent space. The attention map is derived as:

$$A = \sigma(W_a \cdot Z + b_b) \tag{68}$$

where W_a and b_b are learnable weights and biases of the attention network, and $\sigma(\cdot)$ represents the softmax function, ensuring that the attention weights sum to 1 across spatial dimensions, emphasizing the most important regions of the feature map. The attention map is then applied elementwise to the latent representation Z using the Hadamard product (element-wise multiplication):

$$\tilde{Z} = A \odot Z \tag{69}$$

Here, $\tilde{Z} \in \mathbb{R}^{h'xw'xd}$ is the attended latent representation, which retains important features while down-weighting noise. This attended latent space is then passed to the decoder $f_{decoder}(\cdot)$ to reconstruct the denoised image $\hat{X}$:

$$\hat{X} = f_{decoder}(\tilde{Z}) \tag{70}$$

It aims to reduce the disparity between a clean original image and a denoised reconstructed image $\hat{\boldsymbol{X}}$. As a result of training models, the mean squared error (MSE) between the clean image and the denoised image is used, which is defined as follows:

$$L_{mse} = \frac{1}{n} \sum_{i=1}^{n} (X_i - \hat{X}_i)^2 \tag{71}$$

The following step is to introduce an attention regulation term to facilitate the attention mechanism's ability to focus on relevant areas of the image. With this term, the attention map is penalized for excessive diffusion, ensuring the model concentrates on the most salient areas. According to the attention map, regularization is based on the L1 norm as follows:

$$L_{att} = \frac{1}{n}\sum_{i=1}^{n} ||A_i||_1 \quad (72)$$

where,

$||A_i||_1$ is the L1 norm of the attention map for the $i - th$ sample, encouraging sparsity in the attention weights. The final loss function used to train the model combines the reconstruction loss (mean squared error) and the attention regularization:

$$L = L_{mse} + \lambda L_{att} \quad (73)$$

Here, λ determines the trade-off between reconstructing a clean image and sparsely mapping attention. In autoencoding with attention, the autoencoder is trained to minimize compound loss, preserving relevant anatomical structures and eliminating both real and synthetic speckle noise from ultrasound images. This is an important addition to our work as the regularization-based attention mechanism allows the model to distinguish noise and informative features in a better way, resulting in better denoising. The attention mechanism of the proposed AAE model enhances the performance of denoising of the PCOS ultrasound images through selectively enhancing the salient regions and dampening noise. In contrast to the conventional methods of filtering the whole image with a uniform noise reduction, attention-based methods use a network to selectively focus on diagnostically relevant regions, such as ovarian cysts and follicular patterns, and reduce speckle noise. By so doing, it ensures that vital anatomical information is retained, so that it does not lose the delicate structures to make a proper PCOS diagnosis. Moreover, dynamically weighting features with the attention gate network allows the model to learn to differentiate between noise and useful patterns and, therefore, it is less susceptible to over-smoothing. This leads to an increase in image sharpness and diagnostic readability.

Moreover, the attention mechanism provides the model with greater generalizability because it can cope with various levels of noise, and it becomes more robust to various imaging conditions.

4.5.5 Approach to denoising raw PCOS images

Here, an autoencoder is an attention-based denoiser of ultrasound images. The model is able to remove the noise and retain the important features that are useful in detecting PCOS with the aid of the attention mechanism. These methods allow one to adaptively learn the noise pattern to enhance image denoising compared to the currently used methods. Thereafter, the different processes are explained to remove noise:

Step 1: To begin with, gather all the ultrasound images and carry out certain preprocessing actions, i.e. smoothing, normalization, and resizing, which can assist in making the images more comprehensible and improved images. Thereafter, the database is speckled with noise at multiple levels to undergo additional testing.

Step 2: Once this is done, these noisy images are fed into the proposed model to initiate the training. The model is exposed to various noise levels, and therefore, will be able to learn to differentiate between noise and useful features of the image.

Step 3: Select the significant parts of the image to extract features, which are important in noise filtering and in maintaining important details of the image by attention.

Step 4: In order to assess the effectiveness of the image denoising process, this paper will compare the image with state-of-the-art techniques, by assessing its quality, in this case, Structural Similarity Index Measure (SSIM) and Peak Signal-to-Noise Ratio (PSNR). The denoising workflow is summarized in table 4.5.

Table 4.5: Summary of the Denoising Workflow

Step	Operation	Purpose
Step 1	Preprocessing and Noise Addition	To standardize inputs and simulate real-world noise
Step 2	Training with AAE	To learn noise-invariant latent representations
Step 3	Attention-Based Filtering	To enhance key regions and suppress noise adaptively
Step 4	Evaluation using SSIM & PSNR	To assess image quality and compare with baseline models

4.6 METHODOLOGY FOR OBJECTIVE 3:

To develop a deep learning model for testing the accuracy of polycystic ovarian syndrome in ultrasound images

The third objective is achieved in the classification stage, a crucial step in a deep learning-based framework for detecting polycystic ovarian syndrome (PCOS). After ovarian cysts are identified on ultrasound images, the system must evaluate these areas to determine whether the reported ovarian morphology aligns with PCOS or falls within the spectrum of normal variation. This is fundamentally a pattern recognition problem, in which the model distinguishes between normal and PCOS-affected ovaries using extensive annotated data. To fulfill objective 3 in this work, a two-stage framework of deep learning is planned to be used to automate the process of detection and classification of polycystic ovarian syndrome (PCOS) based on ovarian ultrasound images. The model is based on the combination of object detection and image classification to initially identify cysts in the ovary, and then determine whether the ovarian condition is infected or non-infected. In contrast to traditional approaches, which have to be manual cyst countering and subjectively interpreted, this model offers a fully automated, precise, and interpretable diagnosis pipeline. Nonetheless, these images are very difficult to analyze manually because of low contrast, noise, and ovarian structure differences. These are some of the reasons that lead to inconsistencies. Fig. 4.5 below shows the proposed method for detecting and classifying PCOS from ultrasound images. First, images from a dataset undergo preprocessing, including normalization, noise reduction, and reshaping. Data augmentation is also applied to enhance the training data. Later, follicle detection is performed using YOLOv8 in combination with the Attention-Guided Multi-Scale Feature Fusion (AGMSFF) module. The identified regions are subsequently categorized using a ResNet50 model with SE Blocks, which enhances precision by emphasizing critical traits. The system classifies the image as infected or not infected and uses Grad-CAM for interpretability, enabling visualization of the image regions that influenced the classification. The detailed explanation of each is provided below of the above process is as follows:

4.6.1 Classification

In deep learning, classification is a supervised machine learning task where a model categorizes input data into one of several predefined classes or labels. It denotes the process of categorizing input data into established classes based on patterns acquired from training data. The primary objective of the classification is to enable a system to make decisions or predictions when it encounters new, unseen data. In this study, classification is applied to define an abnormal and normal ovary.

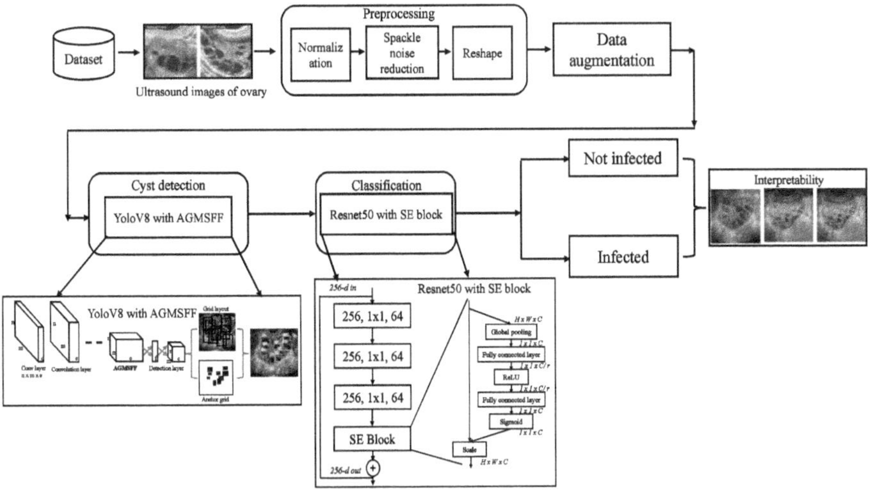

Fig. 4.5: Model prototype for the proposed model for detecting and classifying PCOS using ultrasound images (Pandey et al., 2025a)

As a rule, normal images do not depict any detectable follicles, and abnormal images depict detectable follicles, which is one of the main features of polycystic ovary syndrome (PCOS). Such categorization is essential in making the difference between healthy and those who need additional medical care. In order to solve this challenge of complexity in ultrasound imaging, Squeeze-and-Excitation Blocks (SE-ResNet50) has been suggested as a variation of ResNet50. The ResNet50 network is expanded to include Squeeze-and-Excitation (SE) Blocks after every residual block. The SE dynamically adapts the feature maps to highlight the most informative channels and, as a result, significantly improves the model to distinguish fine differences between normal and pathological ovarian structures. SE block has two phases namely: **Squeeze** and **Excitation**.

For a feature map,

$$\boldsymbol{F} \in \boldsymbol{R}^{H\,x\,W\,x\,C} \tag{74}$$

where $\boldsymbol{H}, \boldsymbol{W}, \boldsymbol{C}$ represent the height, width, and number of channels. The squeeze step computes global context by applying Global Average Pooling (GAP) across spatial dimensions:

$$z_c = \frac{1}{H\,x\,W} \sum_{i=1}^{H} \sum_{j=1}^{W} F_{i,j,c} \tag{75}$$

This produces a channel-wise descriptor $\boldsymbol{z} \in \boldsymbol{R}^{C}$. In the excitation step, fully connected layers with activation functions learn channel-wise dependencies and generate attention weights $\boldsymbol{s}$:

$$\mathbf{s} = \sigma\left(\mathbf{W_2} \cdot \mathbf{RELU}\,(\mathbf{W_1} \cdot \mathbf{z})\right) \tag{76}$$

where, $\boldsymbol{W_1}, \boldsymbol{W_2}$ are learnable weights, and $\boldsymbol{\sigma}$ is the sigmoid activation.

The feature map is recalibrated by scaling each channel with its corresponding weight:

$$F'_{i,j,c} = s_c \cdot F_{i,j,c} \tag{77}$$

This enables the model to highlight essential features, such as cyst-like patterns, while attenuating extraneous irrelevant noise. The altered ResNet50 retrieves features from the ultrasound images, while the SE blocks recalibrate the feature maps at each residual stage. The final layer executes binary classification into normal or abnormal categories, with a SoftMax activation function output:

$$\hat{y} = softmax(W_f \cdot F_{final} + b_f) \tag{78}$$

where,

- $\boldsymbol{W_f}$ and $\boldsymbol{b_f}$ are the weights and bias of the final fully connected layer,
- $\boldsymbol{F_{final}}$ represents the output feature vector.

This integration yields better classification results than existing methodologies. These enhancements render SE-ResNet50 especially well-suited for precise classification of normal and abnormal ovaries in the diagnosis of polycystic ovary syndrome (PCOS).

4.6.2 Interpretability

Interpretability plays a vital role in medical AI in decision-making, especially when it comes to PCOS diagnosis because it has to offer transparent and defensible choices acceptable to doctors and follow logical reasoning. Imposing areas on the ultrasound pictures which is used by a model to arrive at its decision assists in creating confidence and accuracy thus minimizing bias and other irrelevant areas. However, the majority of studies that use the PCOS detection methods are more concerned with the detection error than with the interpretability, and clinical application where explainable results are meaningful. To address this gap, we add Gradient-weighted Class Activation Mapping (Grad-CAM) to localize image areas that contribute to model predictions in addition to enhancing the validity of diagnostics. Grad-CAM works by utilizing the gradients of the output class score y^c with respect to the feature maps A^k of the last convolutional layer. The importance weights α_k^c for each feature map are computed:

$$\alpha_k^c = \frac{1}{Z}\sum_i\sum_j \frac{\partial y^c}{\partial A_{ij}^k} \tag{79}$$

Where Z is the spatial dimension of the feature map, and A_{ij}^k represents the activation at the spatial location (i, j) . The Grad-CAM heatmap L^c is then generated by a weighted combination of the feature maps:

$$L^c = ReLU\left(\sum_k \alpha_k^c A^k\right) \tag{80}$$

The ReLU is used to make sure that only features that positively contribute to the class score are brought out. In order to visualize the decision of the model, the resulting heatmap is superimposed on the initial image. Using Grad-CAM, the system allows clinicians to confirm that the attention of the model matches areas of diagnostic importance, including cysts in abnormal images or homogenous ovarian morphology in normal cases. This extra interpretability would ensure that the classification model is not only accurate but also reliable and clear and thus makes it even more applicable in practical clinical settings.

4.7 CHAPTER SUMMARY

In this chapter, various methodologies have been described which are adopted for the achievement of all the objectives for developing automated PCOS diagnosis using optimized deep learning on ultrasound images. The research structure is logically structured to assure reliability, reproducibility and accuracy in the identification of abnormalities of the ovaries. The chapter has started with a thorough understanding of system design and outlining the steps involved between the acquisition of data and the evaluation of the model. Pre-processing of ultrasound images of ovaries was done to eliminate noise, improve contrast, and equalize the intensity levels to maintain a uniform input quality. Lastly, a discussion of the methodological justifications was given on how each step leads to the attainment of reliable and explainable PCOS detection. The techniques outlined are the basis of the findings and discussion in the next chapter.

CHAPTER-5

RESULT AND DISCUSSION

The chapter provides all experimental findings acquired in the process of developing the two proposed frameworks that aim at solving diagnostic issues related to Polycystic Ovary Syndrome (PCOS) in ultrasound images. The first framework is a noise reduction system in form of Multi-Level Attention Autoencoder (AAE); the other framework is formulated by creating an accurate and interpretable PCOS classification by creating a Dual-Stage Deep Learning Model. With a combination of the two methods, they constitute a well-developed pipeline of enhancing the quality of ultrasound images and gaining a reliable and explainable diagnosis of PCOS.

5.1 SYSTEM DESIGN OVERVIEW

This research's system architecture provides a comprehensive structure for an optimized deep learning technique to detect Polycystic Ovary Syndrome (PCOS) using ultrasound images. The developed system is a well-structured, modular pipeline in which, at each step, a specific task is performed to achieve the research objectives: data collection, image noise removal, and the development of a robust, reliable method for accurate, early detection of PCOS. Thus, as step one, ultrasound images are first collected from various sources and then moved to the preprocessing stage to standardize dimensions and enhance visual quality, facilitating reliable analysis. A controlled speckle noise is then added to the image to provide and simulate a real-world ultrasound imaging scenario. Later, this added noise is processed using the proposed denoising model, i.e., an attention-based autoencoder (AAE), to remove noise and improve the visibility of the follicle in the image. After denoising, the processed images are fed into a deep learning-based classification model, such as a Convolutional Neural

Network (CNN) or an optimized architecture like EfficientNet, for automated detection of polycystic ovarian morphology. Once these have been done the performance evaluation metrics of the system to check the efficacy of the module are accuracy, sensitivity, F1 Score and specificity and the results compared with the current baselines will identify the change that has been made by the proposed system. Such formulated system design also guarantees that all the elements in the image pre-processing process till the concluding classification are integrated in harmony to come up with a strong and trusted PCOS detection system. Fig. 5.1 below gives a summary of the proposed system.

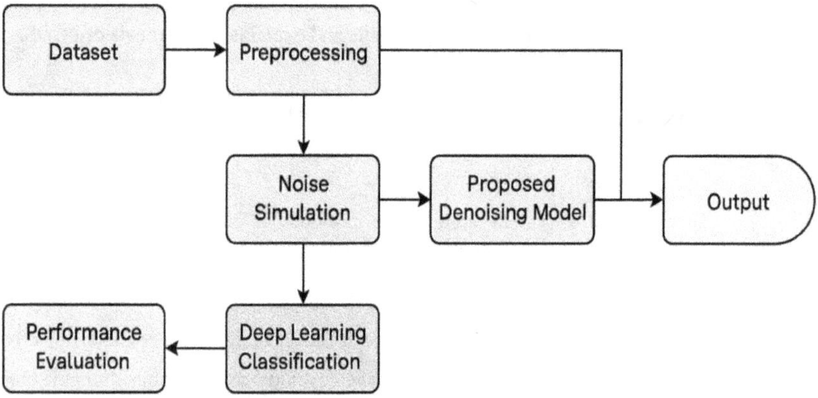

Fig. 5.1 : System Overview

5.2 EXPERIMENTAL SETUP

In Objective 1 and 3: In this thesis, we used two ultrasound image databases that were publicly accessible. The dataset was divided into two after the extraction of features into 2,685 images used as training and 671 images used as testing. It is preceded by follicle detection, classified and then the interpretability analysis. The use of this approach offers a broad account of the capability of the model to locate and classify images particularly in the presence of noise. Comparing with such conditions, this approach will ensure that the model will be efficient in real-life situations.

Objective 2: In the present study, the performance of a given denoising method is evaluated on a publicly availed dataset of 3,356 PCOS ultrasound images. These images have three levels of speckle noise which are 0.001, 0.02 and 0.5. The sample size is 2,685 training images and 671 testing images. The more the noise level is trained in the model, the more it becomes resistant against different types of noise. This plan is a systematic evaluation of the model and its effectiveness in removing noise and successful detection of data in the presence of varying noise levels, which confirms strong functionality in real-world scenarios.

5.3 PERFORMANCE EVALUATION METRICS

In Objectives 1 and 3, the model performance is measured with the help of standard measures. As a performance measure in the context of follicle detection, **mean Average Precision** (mAP) score, which is the level of precision of the model at different recalls, is employed. **Accuracy** (the ratio of correctly categorized instances), **precision** (the ratio of true positives to the predicted positives), **recall** (the proportion of positive instances that are rightly predicted), and **F1-score** (the harmonic mean of precision and recall) are the metrics applied in the context of classification. The results are also visualized by using **ROC-AUC** curve (to demonstrate the trade-off between the true positive rate and false positive rate) and **Confusion Matrix** (to demonstrate the distribution of the predicted and actual classes).

In Objective 2, two metrics that are convenient to measure the performance of the model are **PSNR** and **SSIM**. **PSNR** gives a quantitative value of the image quality following the denoising process by calculating the ratio between the maximum power of an image and the power of the noise that corrupts it. It is computed as:

$$PSNR = 10 \cdot log_{10} \left(\frac{MAX_I^2}{MSE} \right) \tag{81}$$

where,

- $\boldsymbol{MAX_I^2}$ is the maximum pixel value, and
- **MSE** represents the Mean Squared Error between the denoised and clean ultrasound images.

A high value of **PSNR** shows performance of denoising and the nearness of the original image. **SSIM**, in its turn, compares structural similarity between images on the basis of luminance, contrast and structural details. It has a scale between -1 and 1 with a closer value to 1 depicting a similarity.

The **SSIM** is given by:

$$SSIM\ (x, y) = \frac{(2\mu_x\mu_y + C_1)(2\sigma_{xy} + C_2)}{(\mu_x^2 + \mu_y^2 + C_1)(\sigma_x^2 + \sigma_y^2 + C_2)} \tag{82}$$

where,

- $\mu_x\ and\ \mu_y$ are the means,
- $\sigma_x^2\ and\ \sigma_y^2$ are variance
- σ_{xy} is the covariance of images $x\ and\ y$,
- while $C_1\ and\ C_2$ are constants.

Together, **PSNR** and **SSIM** provide a comprehensive evaluation of the denoising models' performance in preserving image fidelity and structural details.

5.4 EXPERIMENTAL RESULTS FOR FOLLICLE DETECTION

For Objective 1 & 3: These results pertain to objectives 1 and 3, in which follicles were detected using different methods, including the proposed method. Fig. 5.2 shows the detection approaches for ovarian follicles in ultrasound images, including OCD-FCNN (Jeevitha & Priya, 2022a). YOLOv8, Attention-Guided Multi-Scale CNN, and the proposed approach. All techniques were benchmarked against ground-truth annotations to assess their efficacy. There is also a model called OCD-FCNN for ovarian follicle detection and classification, which is based on the above index but achieves only 55% mAP. This suggests it may not accurately identify and classify ovarian follicles, leading to incomplete or imprecise predictions.

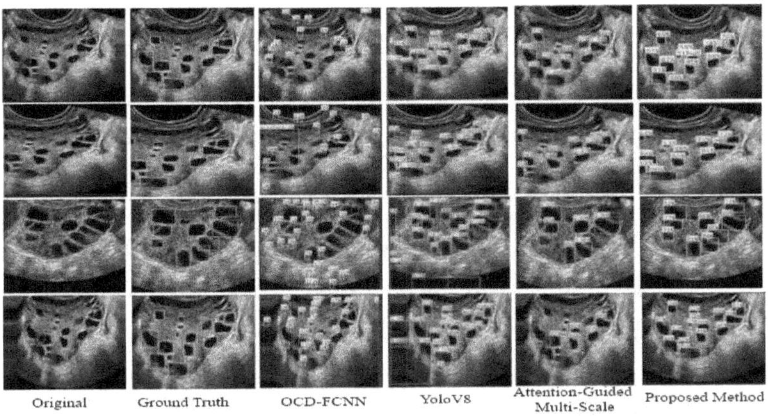

Fig. 5.2 : Detection Result of proposed method along with different state- of- art methods

Even with a 78% mAP, YOLOv8 succeeded in detection but did not identify all targets or achieve comprehensive follicle detection. Similarly, the proposed Attention-Guided Multi-Scale CNN yielded a performance comparable to YOLOv8, indicating that

AMSCNN cannot outperform YOLOv8 in detecting finely nuanced follicle details. The proposed methodology combines an Attention-Guided Multi-Scale CNN with YOLOv8 to improve operational efficiency, leveraging the capabilities of both models to enhance the technique's effectiveness. With an added advantage of a 92% boost in mean Average Precision (mAP), the integration of YOLOv8, an improved object detection algorithm, with the attention-guided mechanism, produces results with a better outcome in terms of detection accuracy and robustness. The proposed methodology demonstrates superior accuracy in localizing ovarian follicles and improves precision and coverage, thereby validating its utility in more complex medical image analysis applications. This follicle detection improves our classification model's performance, enabling it to surpass existing techniques.

For objective 2: The goal is to design a new filtering technique that will be useful in filtering noise in ultrasound images. This goal is met by suggesting an attention-based autoencoder model. The effectiveness of the proposed model was determined as compared to the five available advanced denoising methods i.e. the mean filter, Laplacian filter, bilateral filter, the two-stage picture denoising, and OBNLM filter. In the process of noise removal, each of the methods plays a different role: the mean filter averages the pixel values whereas the Laplacian filter sharpens the edges and the bilateral filter maintains the edges. Two-stage Image denoising method employs Discrete Wavelet Transform (DWT) to break and threshold wavelets and a neural network to classify noise patterns so that they can be used to adaptively filter. Combined with a CNN, the OBNLM filter is useful in removing speckle noise, resulting in a smooth, denoised image. All these methods together create a complete system of ultrasound image denoising. Table 5.1 indicates the effectiveness of various techniques in removing noise at various levels (At a variance level of 0.5, the recommended technique will give a PSNR of 31.33, which is significantly higher than the existing techniques and an improvement of 7% over the second bilateral filter PSNR of 29.32). The proposed method achieves a PSNR of 34.25 and an SSIM of

92.33 at a lower variance of 0.02, which is 7.5 percent better than the next best OBNLM filter (30.98 PSNR).

Table 5.1 Proposed denoised method with state-of-the-art techniques performance evaluation metrics

	Performance after denoise					
Performance before denoise	**0.5**		**0.02**		**0.001**	
Performance metric	PSNR	SSIM	PSNR	SSIM	PSNR	SSIM
Mean filter (Kiruthika et al., 2020)	28.31	15.63	28.40	45.91	28.52	54.28
Laplacian filter (Choubey et al., 2021)	28.35	18.23	28.49	55.25	28.46	60.80
Bilateral (Coupé et al., 2009)	29.32	30.23	29.65	60.25	29.74	72.19
Two-Stage Denoising (Jha et al., 2024)	29.35	48.52	29.72	67.32	29.83	78.54
OBNLM Filter (Vasavi et al., 2020)	29.40	60.80	30.98	88.24	31.22	89.76
Proposed Method	**31.33**	**85.21**	**34.25**	**92.33**	**36.23**	**99.25**

The suggested approach achieves a PSNR of 36.23 and a remarkable SSIM of 99.25 for the lowest noise variance (0.001), demonstrating a significant SSIM improvement over the OBNLM filter, which attained an SSIM of 89.76. The suggested approach also shows superior outcomes as it is based on an attention-driven autoencoder framework that can successfully detect and retain fine details of images and concentrate on denoising areas. Unlike the old-fashioned methods such as the mean and Laplacian filters, both of which are restricted by their straight forward nature, the mean filter has the disadvantage of smoothing out vital information by averaging pixel values and as such the Laplacian filter, which is mainly used to detect edges, enhances noise. The bilateral filter is effective in maintaining edges, but is not very good with the noise level. Two stage image denoising technique tends to over smooth the image at the cost of detail in the process of removing noise. Unlike these approaches, the suggested attention-based autoencoder optimistically enhances the quality of an image and demonstrates particular benefits at all noise levels considered.

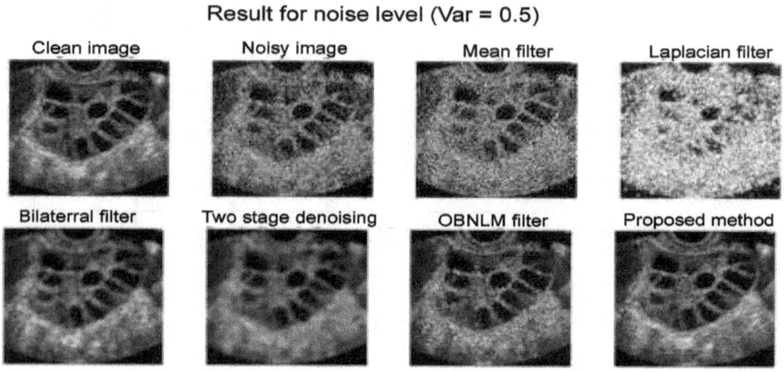

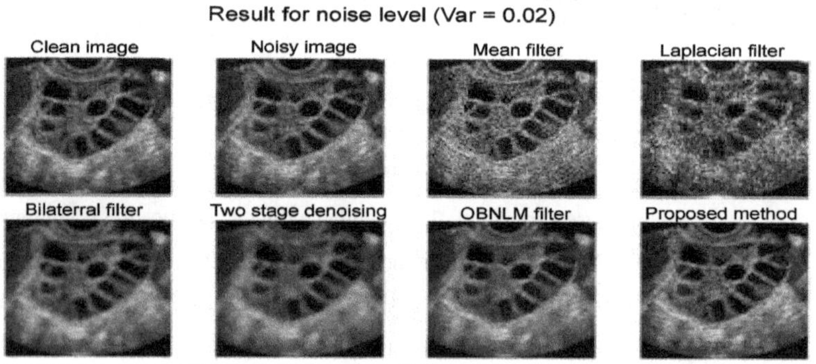

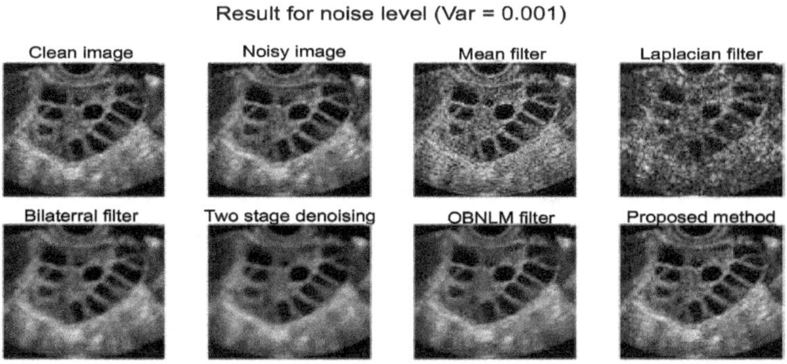

Fig. 5.3 : Qualitative results of at different variance noise levels during the denoising process

At noise variances of 0.5, 0.02, and 0.001, Fig. 5.3 shows the performance of various denoising methods on an ultrasound image. The noisy image is extremely grainy, making it challenging to discern structural details. As per the study done, at the highest noise level where variance level 0.5, some filters like the mean and bilateral filters manage to reduce noise but they often blur essential characteristics and the Laplacian filter emphasizes edges but fails to address noise effectively at this high level where as the OBNLM filter and the two-stage image denoising technique attains an average level of noise reduction, but only the proposed method effectively removes around all most noise while not hampering the other characteristics of the image, hence resulting in the clearest output even in challenging noise condition. As the noise variance level decreases to 0.02 and then 0.001, all methods show improved results, containing structural details that are also visible in the image. At a variance level of 0.02, filters such as OBNLM and bilateral filters provide greater clarity while reducing noise, but blurring and minor artifacts still persist. By the time the variance level reaches 0.001, the denoising methods begin producing images that are quite close to the originals. Finally, the proposed methodology is superior to others at all noise levels and provides the cleanest images with the best structural fidelity, indicating its strength and flexibility to the changing noise conditions. Fig. 5.4 provides the comparison of the performance of the current denoising methods and the proposed one regarding various.

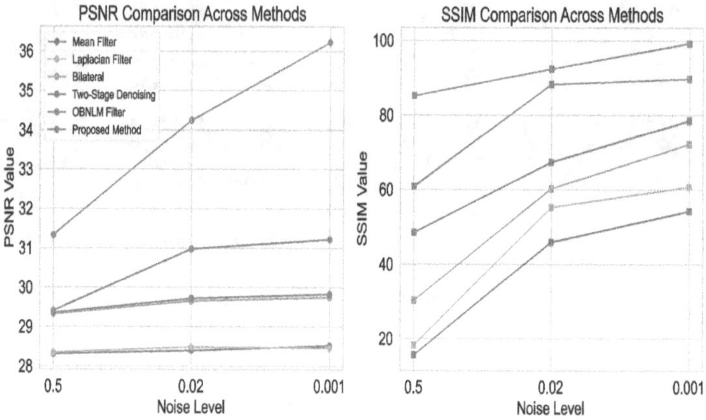

Fig. 5.4 : Based on PSNR(Left) and SSIM(Right) Across Different Noise Levels, a Comparison of existing denoising methods with the proposed methods

noise levels, using the PSNR and SSIM parameters. In both graphs, noise levels are shown on the horizontal axis, with lower values indicating less noise, and PSNR and SSIM values are shown on the vertical axis. The higher the PSNR and SSIM values, the better the image quality after denoising. The proposed method outperforms traditional methods across all noise levels, achieving the highest PSNR and SSIM values, demonstrating better image quality than methods such as the mean filter, the Laplacian filter, the bilateral filter, the OBNLM Filter, and two-stage denoising. The other methods show average improvisation at even lower noise levels but are still less effective than the proposed methodology. Fig. 5.5 illustrates the performance of various denoising techniques across different noise levels using a radar chart. In the chart, an axis is shown for each noise level (0.5, 0.02, and 0.001), with the higher value on each axis indicating improved performance in retaining image quality during denoising. The proposed method outperforms other methods across all noise levels, as indicated by its broader spread across the chart. There are other techniques, including the mean filter, the Laplacian filter, the bilateral filter, the two-stage denoising, and the OBNLM filter, with lesser spreads, revealing lower PSNR and SSIM values and hence less efficient denoising. The radar chart shows clearly that the Proposed Method is better in meeting similarities in structures and signal-to-noise ratio in different noise levels.

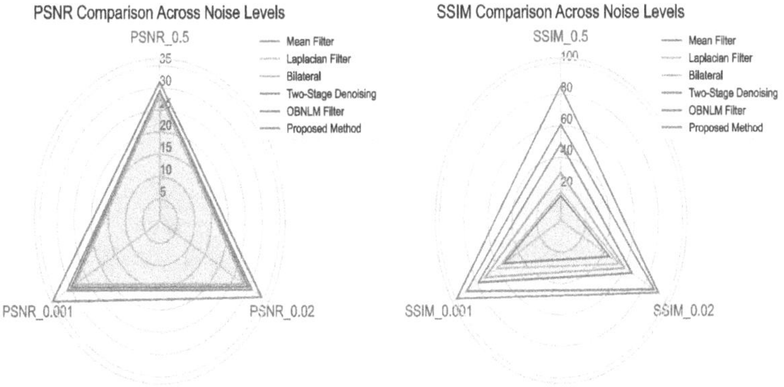

Fig. 5.5 : Comparison of denoising methods and proposed method based on PSNR and SSIM across different noise levels

5.5 EXPERIMENTAL RESULTS FOR CLASSIFICATION

For objectives 1 and 3, the suggested classification method proves to be exceptionally effective, with the best accuracy on both Dataset 1 and Dataset 2, as can be seen in Table 5.2. It achieved 98.25 on Dataset1, which is better than ResNet50 (95.69%), DenseNet121 (92.87%), and VGG16 (89.26%). The addition of Squeeze-and-Excitation (SE) blocks significantly enhanced all the baseline models with DenseNet121 attaining accuracy of 94.65% (an improvement of 92.87) and VGG16 attaining accuracy of 91.33% (an improvement of 89.26). In the same way, the proposed method achieved 94.56 on Dataset2, which is higher than ResNet50 (90.21%), DenseNet121 (84.33%), and VGG16 (85.66%). SE blocks were found to be more effective at feature representation, which allowed models to learn finer data patterns and generalize more. This resulted in an improvement of 2.56% over ResNet50 and 3.6% over DenseNet121 (with SE blocks) on Dataset 1, as well as an improvement of 4.35 and 4.45 on Dataset 2, respectively. These findings confirm that SE blocks recalibrate channel-wise responses to emphasize important features, which is a development in the state of the art in classification tasks.

Table 5.2 : Performance evaluation of proposed classification method with state-of-the-art methods

Dataset	Models	Accuracy (%)	Precision (%)	Recall (%)	F1-Score (%)
Dataset1	Vgg16	89.26	90.33	89.65	89.98
	Resnet50	95.69	94.12	96.74	95.41
	Densenet121	92.87	93.79	91.55	92.65
	Vgg16 with SE Blocks	91.33	90.12	91.54	90.82
	Densenet121 with SE blocks	94.65	95.47	94.66	95.06
	Resnet50 with SE blocks (Proposed Method)	**98.25**	**97.65**	**98.66**	**98.15**
Dataset2	Vgg16	85.66	86.78	85.12	85.94
	Resnet50	90.21	89.33	88.32	88.82
	Densenet121	84.33	85.63	84.11	84.86
	Vgg16 with SE Blocks	88.25	89.44	88.14	88.78
	Densenet121 with SE blocks	90.11	88.25	86.32	87.27
	Resnet50 with SE blocks (Proposed Method)	**94.56**	**92.32**	**93.55**	**92.93**

The following Fig. 5.6 shows the training and validation accuracies of the proposed model on two datasets; the left plot corresponds to the first dataset, while the right plot corresponds to the second. The blue hue in each plot denotes the training accuracy, whereas the orange hue signifies the validation accuracy. The model shows rapid growth in the first epochs, then gradually converges to optimal accuracy as the number of epochs increases. The training and validation accuracies are equally high, so the model may be considered to generalize well, with little risk of overfitting.

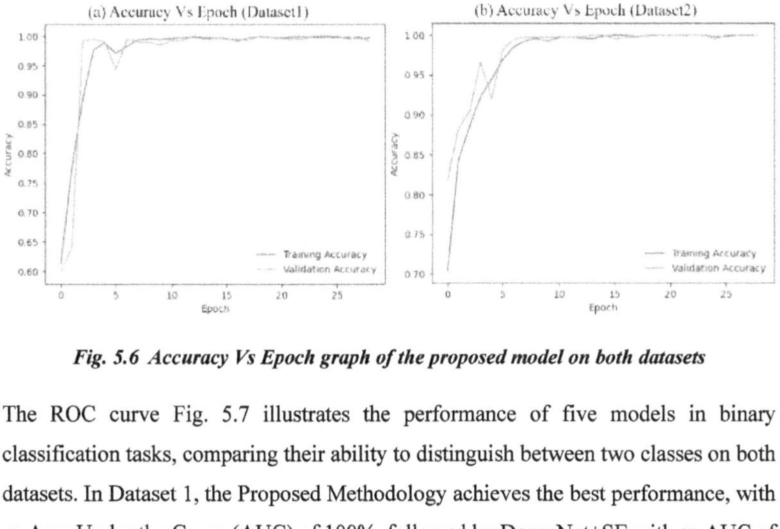

Fig. 5.6 Accuracy Vs Epoch graph of the proposed model on both datasets

The ROC curve Fig. 5.7 illustrates the performance of five models in binary classification tasks, comparing their ability to distinguish between two classes on both datasets. In Dataset 1, the Proposed Methodology achieves the best performance, with an Area Under the Curve (AUC) of 100%, followed by DenseNet+SE with an AUC of 98%. VGG16 and ResNet50 perform moderately well, each with an AUC of 88%, while DenseNet has a slightly lower AUC of 85%. In Dataset 2, the proposed method achieves an AUC of 92%, indicating its generalizability. A curve's proximity to the top-left corner indicates superior model performance, with all models outperforming random guessing (represented by the diagonal line). This demonstrates the Proposed Method's superiority in classification accuracy compared to the others.

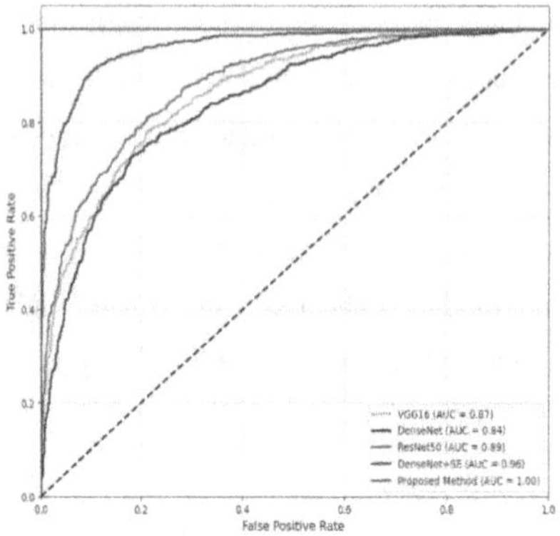

(a) ROC curve Dataset 1

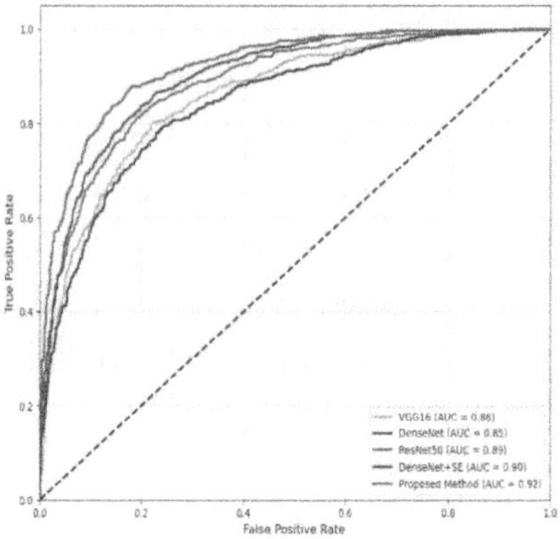

(a) ROC curve Dataset 2

Fig. 5.7 ROC curve of the proposed method along with other methods on both datasets.

Table 5.3 below compares the performance of existing techniques with that of the proposed model across two datasets in terms of accuracy. For Dataset 1, previous methods, such as Nilofer et al., 2021 (Nilofer & Ramkumar, 2021) got 97.50%, Gopalakrishnan et al., 2021 (Gopalakrishnan & Iyapparaja, 2020) got 93.83%, Rachana et al., 2021 (Rachana et al., 2021b) got 97.00%, and Moral et al., 2024 (Moral, Mustafi, & Sahana, 2024) got 96.54%, demonstrating high accuracy, but the proposed method surpasses it with 98.25%, showcasing its superior performance. Similarly, for Dataset 2, existing techniques like Nakhua et al., 2024 (Nakhua et al., 2024) got 92.00%, Poonam Moral et al., 2024 (Moral, Mustafi, & Sahana, 2024) for 94.39%, and Lakshmi et al., 2023 (Lakshmi et al., 2023) For 91.07%, the method achieves notable accuracy, but the proposed method achieves the highest accuracy at 94.56%. The results demonstrate the superiority of the suggested model over leading methodologies across several datasets.

Table 5.3 Performance evaluation of proposed classification methods with existing methods.

Dataset	Models	Accuracy (%)
Dataset 1	Nilofer et al. 2021 (Nilofer & Ramkumar, 2021)	97.50
	Gopalakrishnan et al. 2021 (Gopalakrishnan & Iyapparaja, 2020)	93.83
	Rachana et al. 2021(Rachana et al., 2021b)	97.00
	Moral et al. 2024 (Moral, Mustafi, Mustafi, et al., 2024b)	96.54
	Proposed Method	**98.25**
Dataset 2	Nakhua et al. 2024 (Nakhua et al., 2024)	92.00
	Moral et al. 2024 (Moral, Mustafi, Mustafi, et al., 2024a)	94.39
	Lakshmi et al. 2023 (Lakshmi et al., 2023)	91.07
	Proposed Method	**94.56**

5.6 EXPERIMENTAL RESULTS FOR INTERPRETABILITY

Deep learning requires interpretability especially in medical imaging tasks such as ultrasound analysis to make the decision made by the model transparent and clinically sound. Fig. 5.8 shows that the proposed model can be interpreted with the help of Grad-CAM applied on the final layer of the network. Grad-CAM can be used to justify the behavior of the model, such as by visualizing the region of focus in the image, and make sure that the predictions of the model are consistent with human expert knowledge, which is important to build trust and improve decision-making in sensitive areas. Grad-CAM has been popular as a technique of producing visual explanations of a model prediction. It points out the areas in the input image that exert the greatest effect on the decision made by the model. Calculating the gradients of the predicted class score with the feature maps of a particular layer, Grad-CAM creates a heatmap that superimposes the original image, highlighting the regions of the highest importance. The grayscale ultrasound images have been provided in the upper row of the figure. By comparison the Grad-CAM visualizations below the bottom row show areas of interest (e.g. cysts or abnormalities) in color-coded heatmaps, with warmer (more important) to cooler (less important) colours. These visualizations ensure that the model is robust and interpretable since the visualizations are able to highlight the diagnostically relevant structures.

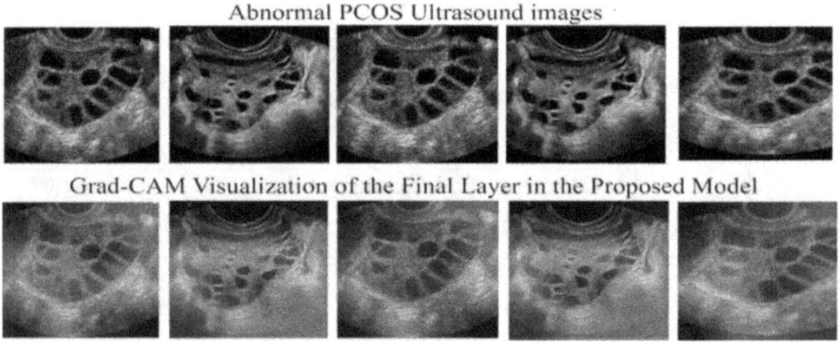

Fig. 5.8 Interpretability of the proposed classification model on different images

5.7 DISCUSSION

This study attempts to categorize PCOS using ultrasound images, as the quality of the images could not be clear and the nature of the disease. The past methods have the drawback that the follicle is not identified and the feature set is inadequate to detect the follicles. To cope with this, we introduce a YOLOv8-based attention-guided multiscale to detect follicles in order to have a better understanding of particular regions of interest and make the input more informative to the classifier. The classification phase involves a ResNet-50 with SE blocks to improve the representation of the features and concentration on the most significant ones. This is a biological prediction system in two stages which significantly enhances the rehabilitative model. Moreover, interoperability is one of the objectives of the model, which may be essential in the process of deep learning-based medical image analysis. It therefore makes sure that the detection of the follicles is included and also offers the practitioners the explanation of the classification results. The reason why this method would be effective is not only that it increases accuracy, but it also gets into the gaps that are present in the current methodology by setting up efficient and highly interpretable detection as the ultimate standard towards PCOS assessment in ultrasound images. However, the offered model has a number of disadvantages. In the detection phase, the proposed YOLOv8 attention-guided multiscale model can be unable to adopt tiny or poorly discernible follicle candidates in low-quality ultrasound images, potentially restricting its use in a wider range of clinical contexts. During the classification phase, SE blocks are added into the ResNet50 network to enhance the network capacity to learn features; nevertheless, it makes the network more expensive to compute. It renders training and inference considerably slower than full accuracy; it restricts the use of the model in real-time applications or devices with a small computational power. Such constraints provide us with thoughts on how to improve them that can be directed at making such systems more practical.

5.8 CHAPTER SUMMARY

The chapter included the entire findings of the design, implementation, and evaluation of the suggested deep learning system to detect PCOS in ultrasound images automatically. The chapter started with the system design overview and layer by layer description of the model architecture, and how the attention based autoencoder and the CNN classifier were organized to aid in noise elimination and accurate classification. After that, all training and hyperparameter consideration was presented in detail, including specific aspects of data preprocessing, optimization methods, and augmentation techniques to provide strong model convergence. Within the performance assessment, the suggested approaches are outlined and assessed in terms of PSNR, SSIM, accuracy, sensitivity, specificity, and F1-score, which provide the reliability of the model both in image denoising and in clinical decisions. The proposed method has been proved to be better at all parameters than the current methods and hence reflect the novelty and the contribution to the medical imaging field. Also, Grad-CAM visualizations combined with it enhanced the model interpretability. Finally, the suggested methodology offers a very reliable, precise, and interpretative deep learning model of PCOS detection, which will be the basis of its further introduction into clinical practice and possible validation studies. The chapter forms a powerful basis to the next chapter that draws the summary and findings of this study.

CHAPTER-6

SUMMARY AND CONCLUSION

6.1 SUMMARY OF FINDINGS

The main objective behind this research is to develop an optimized deep learning technique to detect polycystic ovary syndrome. The goal of this research is obtained by following several key steps, which are: 1) data collection, 2) preparation for future analysis, 3) addressing speckle noise, 4) cleaning the image noise, 5) extracting key features, and then 6) classifying those features. The major findings of this research are summarized as follows :

i. **Image Analysis preparation:** Preprocessing and denoising techniques: preparing the Image analysis by correcting the standard dimensions of the ultrasound images to 128x 128 x 3 was indeed useful in training the model. The attention-based autoencoder (AAE) that the authors developed in the study showed better results in denoising and effective elimination of the speckle noise of the picture without losing finer details of the follicle.

ii. **Incomprehensive and powerful deep learning-based polycystic ovary syndrome (PCOS) classification :** A combination of Attention-based Autoencoder (AAE) and Convolutional Neural Network (CNN) architecture demonstrated high accuracy, sensitivity, and specificity and was able to accurately classify ovarian images of people with and without PCOS. The model strength and consistency were defined and validated based on assessment measures, which were accuracy, F1-score, ROC-AUC, PSNR, and SSIM.

iii. **The comparison analysis between proposed and existing models:** Compared to the current CNN technologies and the traditional autoencoders, the proposed methodology demonstrated superior and enhanced results. This means that it may be applicable in clinical facilities.

iv. **Clinical significance of the proposed method:** The predictions generated by a robust model in the study based on the proposed technique in the form of Grad-CAM heatmaps are of clinical significance since the ovarian structures have been indicated. The findings have validated a better deep learning model, which boosts the errors to a great extent.

6.2 RESEARCH CONTRIBUTIONS

This research is a major step forward in the use of artificial intelligence in medical imaging with the focus on the automated diagnosis of Polycystic Ovary Syndrome (PCOS) using ultrasound images. The study is primarily achieved by the generation of a new, universal deep learning system. In this case, both convolutional neural networks (CNNs) and attention-based autoencoders (AAE) are applied simultaneously, and denoising is carried out. The two-step process combats the issues of ultrasound imaging like the noise of speckles and sensitive follicular patterns and enhances image quality and diagnostic accuracy. This combination of the denoising and classification into one, simplified process in this study offers a powerful, efficient method of the correct and early identification of PCOS. This approach is different compared to the traditional methods that involve a single step. Other factors are the standardization and innovation of ultrasonic image preprocessing. In this case, there involves a structured preparation pipeline that involves image scaling, normalization, noise simulations control and denoising. These few stages were developed to assist the model to cope with image variability in a clinical ultrasonography scan. This improvement renders the proposed solution more trustworthy in practice imaging cases. These scenarios tend to exhibit a very broad variety of contrast, clarity and noise depending on the ultrasound equipment and their operator. The comprehensive evaluation and benchmarking of the model is another key contribution and an important part of the study. The performance of the framework was assessed in detail with the help of a variety of classification and image-quality indicators, such as accuracy, sensitivity, specificity, F1-score, AUC, PSNR, and SSIM. This detailed study gives strong reasoning about why the model has been shown to perform better than the normal CNNs and classical autoencoders. With variability in attention processes and hyperparameters, the proposed model can be more diagnostic in a clinical context as demonstrated by the achieved performance improvement. Moreover, the research will make a considerable contribution to developing reliable and understandable artificial intelligence in the healthcare sector. The results of the study indicate that the model when trained with the class-gradation-weighted activation mapping (Grad-CAM) to predict PCOM identifies the areas that are clinically relevant, including small peripheral follicles and distended ovarian stroma. This ability to visual picture interpretations will instil confidence in physicians regarding AI predictions, which will be the basis of moral and proper application of AI in gynaecology. Besides, the research forms a basis on which more and broader medical uses can be extended and changed. The proposed methodology that encompasses the best method to make data ready, pay attention to the key aspects, and place data into clear categories can be used as the basis of the future research in the field of reproductive health imaging and other diagnostic issues that are associated with ultrasound. With its provision of a clinically relevant and technically sound, yet understandable approach, this study will assist in closing the gap between the research on artificial intelligence and its application to clinical environments.

6.3 LIMITATION OR CONSTRAINTS

Although this research came up with the promising findings, there are several limitations that should be mentioned to give the complete picture of the research. Such a method is limited by the absence of other clinical or biochemical indicators, although ultrasonography may be a primary non-invasive method of diagnosis. As a result, full screenings of polycystic ovarian syndrome (PCOS) do not provide the data on the LH/FSR, indicators of insulin resistance, and testosterone. The integration of imaging and laboratory testing diagnostics techniques in clinical settings may result into more comprehensive and realistic predictions. Improved computation is still required by the model to hardware supporting the use of the model, although in both training and operation of a GPU. Since the model involves the use of high-performance computing resources, it might be difficult to implement in healthcare facilities in poor or isolated regions. To reduce this problem and allow its extensive application in clinical practice, there is a requirement of lighter optimization or edge deployment strategies. Although the Grad-CAM heatmaps can result in a better understanding of the model and induce more confidence in the model predictions, clinical trials are necessary to test its diagnostic accuracy and compliance with the regulations. They identify areas of improvement to ensure that the models are able to move out of the experimental phase to the clinical practice.

6.4 ETHICAL CONSIDERATIONS

Ethics should be considered in the research on artificial intelligence and medical imaging. Preservation of quality of healthcare, patient rights, and privacy and the development of technology are their main objectives. The ethical standards were followed in this work by the means of the data collection, the development and assessment of the model, in order to comply with the biomedical research standards. Anonymisation of all ultrasound images was done in both training and testing, to avoid the retention and storage of patient-identifying information. This method kept the patients confidential and acted as a guarantor of ethical standard in exploiting medical information. The informed consent was guaranteed by getting a dataset available in publicly accessible sources or organizations that had the relevant ethical approval. The patient information will be treated in an ethical manner and all those whose photos had been used in the study will be aware of the potential applications. Moreover, the AI system that was created in the current work was meant to aid the diagnosis but not substitute the judgment of human beings. The model can help gynaecologists and radiologists better identify PCOS cases; however, the ultimate decision concerning the case remains a matter of qualified medical practitioners, which leads to ethical issues regarding the possibility of artificial intelligence to take over the human decision. Another ethical theory looked at the impartiality and biasness of artificial intelligence model. Medical AI systems trained using a small or a failing diverse dataset might fail to work effectively with different groups of patients. This might unwittingly result in unfair diagnosis. The paper notes that there is a need to have unbiased and fair clinical validation of the model in different centres and demographic groups regardless of the high accuracy of the model. This study meets global ethical standards of AI in healthcare since it honours the privacy of the patient, informed consent is obtained, human supervision exists, and it also recognizes the significance of fairness and transparency. These aspects also make the system more reliable as the ground is set to use it in a responsible manner in the clinical setting in the future.

6.5 FUTURE WORK

The positive outcomes of the given study suggest that there are various ways to enhance and optimize the offered AI framework and make it more applicable in a clinical environment. Future studies ought to focus on the extension and modification of the dataset. Although the research found great results, its small sample size and a restricted area of conduct might restrict the models to a wider sample of individuals utilizing ultrasound machines and imaging techniques. The collaboration with diagnostic and medical centers in various locations should be considered in future studies. Considering that this research is more extensive, it will allow addressing a more diverse dataset. These initiatives will produce consistent outcomes in clinical practice through better reliability of the model and decreased assumptions. The combination of diagnosis data of multiple sources is one of the key aspects that should be explored in future studies. Although the study adopted purely ultrasound imaging, integration of imaging outcomes with biochemical, hormonal, and clinical outcomes may result in a more comprehensive diagnostic method. This would comprise of the medical history of the patient, symptoms of insulin resistance and testosterone/FSH ratio. The combination of several strategies would enhance the clinical utility and predictive capability of the model. It is of particular significance in borderline or atypical instances of PCOS since the results of ultrasound may not be sufficient to give a definite diagnosis. Moreover, it can be implemented in the research aimed at the development of a lightweight and real-time AI model that is specifically oriented at portable ultrasound machines and edge devices. Specifically, in isolated regions that have little access to skilled radiologists or in medical facilities, where funding is limited, such models could provide diagnostic support at the place of care. Information distillation, model trimming, and quantization can greatly decrease computational needs with no diagnostic accuracy loss, technically. The validation studies and clinical trials that are conducted in the real hospitals should be introduced in the future research. The incorporation of the AI systems into the routine diagnostic processes will allow the ongoing assessment of the model, the input of physicians, and the control of the regulations. These factors determine the successful implementation and clinical application of the system. Moreover, improving the interpretability of the model using advanced visualization tools in lieu of GRAD-CAM, like layer-wise feature highlighting, can be more useful and increase clinical confidence. This research can be the basis of the development of AI solutions in the field of reproductive health diagnostics. The framework can become a hybrid AI-Assisted reproductive health platform by extending the approach to other related gynaecological issues, such as ovarian cysts, endometriosis, and follicular monitoring in fertility therapies. These future projects are targeted at the connection of experimental AI work to the real-life application in a clinic. Its aim is to develop early and comprehensive and affordable diagnostic tools on global women health.

6.6 REACHING SUSTAINABILITY TARGETS OF SUSTAINABILITY GOALS

This research is a great contribution towards the United Nations Sustainable Development Goals (SDGs) especially those that concern innovation, health, gender equality, and responsible consumer behaviour. The sustainability goals are supported by the two research projects that use deep learning at two phases to detect PCOS and remove noise during ultrasound pictures.

Sustainable Development Goal (SDG 3) Good Health and Well-Being : Early and accurate diagnosis of PCOS, i.e., improving picture quality, accuracy of detection, and classification, is one of the SDG 3 attained in this study. The proposed solutions provide early, dependable, and less biased diagnosis of PCOS. This makes the provision of timely medical care possible. The variations could be due to the fact that there was a high dependency on competence of radiologists in the traditional diagnosis. This method reduces such errors by using explainable classification and attention methods when doing the denoising. As such, it enhances the patient outcomes and effectiveness of healthcare delivery. Ultrasound is not as costly as MRIs or CT scans and thus improving its accuracy with artificial intelligence will mean that high-quality reproductive care is made available in low- and middle-income countries (LMICs) to foster global health equity.

Sustainable Development Goal 5 (SDG5) aims at the realization of gender equality: The health issues of women must be considered. Polycystic ovarian syndrome (also referred to as the PCOS disorder) primarily presents itself in women of reproductive age. The improved diagnostic support systems aid the doctors in treating the condition and this enhances the reproductive health services of women. AI solutions that are reliable and easily understandable ensure an increase in trust between doctors and patients. Grad-CAM enables women to know more about their healthcare options by visualizing the diagnostic process. This philosophy is compatible with the idea of healthcare as something high-quality that would be accessible to everyone.

Sustainable Development Goals SDG 9 of the Industry, Innovation, and Infrastructure: The advancement of technology and processes has fundamentally changed the way we diagnose and treat diseases, and does so using more efficient and accurate image-processing technologies. The outcomes of these developments are improved patient outcomes, accurate diagnosis, and improved healthcare systems. As an example, medical imaging with the help of machine learning and artificial intelligence can help radiologists spot problems much faster and more accurately, classify image abnormalities more simply, and reveal clinical uses of AI-enhanced imaging technology. Moreover, advanced imaging technologies like molecular imaging and functional MRI have helped us learn more about diseases, as they allow us take a deeper look at the functioning of the human body and the development of the disease. Medical imaging is also more available through advancement of portable imaging technology. They are also usually easier to use and carry around and allow photography in remote locations or during emergencies, collect essential diagnostic information, and improve patient care. These advances in medical imaging are broadening the medical field all things being equal. The outcomes of these advances in the diagnosis and treatment of illnesses are better patient outcomes and more efficient healthcare systems. The latest trends in medical imaging have included the application of dual-stage interpretable deep learning to classify and focus on attention-based autoencoders to minimize noise, which has created a flexible and scalable smart healthcare infrastructure that is applicable to both urban and rural hospitals. This paper tackles the black-box issue of AI that has included interpretability that enhances the adaptability of AI in clinical settings and promotes industry-academia partnership in medical AI, which contributes to the innovation infrastructure.

Sustainable Development Goals 10 - Reduced Inequalities: Advanced diagnostic systems are common in urban areas that are rich in resources. Through the measurement of improving the reliability of readily available ultrasound equipment, there will be a way of closing the divide and providing a more equitable delivery of healthcare in rural communities, which in many cases, does not have adequate resources. Global relevance is one of these factors. PCOS is a female condition that can be found anywhere in the world and that is why the recommended techniques can be practiced everywhere. This leads to lessening the health difference between the developed and developing areas.

Sustainable Development Goals 12 - Responsible Consumption and Production: Misdiagnosis may sometimes lead to invasive surgery, unnecessary hormone treatment, or repeated x-ray, ultrasound, or other imaging tests. The proposed frameworks do not require medical procedures that are not necessary and ensure the efficient use of resources and sustainable medical practice through enhancing accuracy and reduction of noise in the first ultrasound scans.

Sustainable Development Goal 17 - centres on the creation of partnerships in order to reach the other objectives: The application of publicly available datasets in both papers is evidence of commitment to open science and sharing of knowledge. This promotes Sustainable Development Goal 17 in that it promotes international collaboration on medical AI research to advance healthcare diagnosis of women in most world states.

6.6 FINAL CONCLUSION

The thesis discussion involves developing an improved deep learning model to determine Polycystic Ovary Syndrome (PCOS) using ultrasound images, which would be a progressive development in applying artificial intelligence to reproductive health care. This emerged methodology is useful in solving the major problems that are experienced during ultrasound diagnosis and they include failure to perceive follicles, speckle noise and precise and accurate automated classification. The given comprehensive study expounds on the possible clinical practice benefits and the application of advanced artificial intelligence tools to identify polycystic ovarian syndrome (PCOS). The PSNR and SSIM scores of image quality and diagnostic performance of such measures as accuracy, sensitivity, specificity, F1-score, and AUC indicate that the new technology is superior to traditional CNNs and autoencoders The methodology entails a powerful Convolutional Neural Network (CNN) classifier and an attention-based autoencoder (AAE) to clean up picture, which yield clearly correct diagnoses, improved image quality, and explainable results on the subject matter in a clinical setting. This research paper concentrates on the significance of AI-assisted early detection on the patient outcomes. Since a late diagnosis of PCOS may cause numerous other chronic conditions, such as heart-related disorders, infertility, ovarian cancer, etc., the proposed strategy may also enhance the overall level of services provided by gynaecologists and radiologists. It aims to standardize assessments and minimize diagnostic delays by offering an easy, effective, and interpretable diagnostic tool. The positive outcomes of the study provide new possibilities to apply clinical applications and develop the effective real-time artificial intelligence tools, combined diagnostic models, and shared data across multiple centres.

6.7 CHAPTER SUMMARY

This chapter presents all the aspects of the research and includes the most important conclusions, contributions, limitations, ethical issues and recommendations. The deep learning-based innovative technology depicts an impressive breakthrough in respect of detecting Polycystic ovary syndrome among the ultrasound images promptly and efficiently. The authors have done this wonderful breakthrough by the combination of a convolutional neural network (CNN) which is used in classification and an attention-based autoencoder (AAE) which is used in noise reduction. Conversely, the interpretability has been made possible by the GRAD-CAM visualization and it shows the model has excellent performance in terms of high accuracy, sensitivity and interpretability. This is an indicator that the technology that has been developed is therapeutically sound and technically sound. Further directions of this research are also discussed in the use of multimodal data, creation of more effective model variations, and comprehensive clinical evaluations. The study is an essential step towards a trustworthy, sound, and convenient AI-facilitated reproductive healthcare system, also achieving the several UN Sustainable Development Goals. It has a tangible basis on future advancements in the diagnostics of women health.